# TESTOSTERONE IS YOUR FRIEND

## Other Health Books by Roger Mason

*Lower Blood Pressure Without Drugs*

*Lower Your Cholesterol Without Drugs*

*Macrobiotics for Everyone*

*Natural Health for Women*

*No More Horse Estrogen!*

*The Minerals You Need*

*The Natural Diabetes Cure*

*The Natural Prostate Cure*

*The Supplements You Need*

*What is Beta Glucan?*

# TESTOSTERONE IS YOUR FRIEND

## A Book for Men and Women

## ROGER MASON

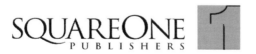

SQUAREONE
PUBLISHERS

*Testosterone Is Your Friend* is not intended as medical advice. It is written solely for informational and educational purposes. Please consult a health professional should the need for one be indicated. Because there is always some risk involved, the author and publisher are not responsible for any adverse effects or consequences resulting from the use of any of the suggestions, preparations, or methods described in the book. The publisher does not advocate the use of any particular diet or health program, but believes the information presented in this book should be available to the public.

COVER DESIGNER: Jeannie Tudor
IN-HOUSE EDITOR: Ally Cirruzzo
TYPESETTER: Gary A. Rosenberg

**Square One Publishers**
115 Herricks Road
Garden City Park, NY 11040
(516) 535-2010 • (877) 900-BOOK
www.squareonepublishers.com

**Library of Congress Cataloging-in-Publication Data**

Printed in the United States of America

10   9   8   7   6   5   4   3   2   1

# Contents

# About This Book

*This is the most comprehensive, researched, factual, and effective book about testosterone for men and women in the world.* Testosterone is not a Magic Hormone, to be used by itself, to cure what ails you. All our hormones work together harmoniously in concert, and all of them must be balanced together as a team. Chapter 17, "Your Other Hormones," is the most important one to read. Our hormones are basic and vital to our health and wellbeing. Hormone imbalance is one of the factors in all illnesses.

Men should read my *The Natural Prostate Cure,* and women should read my *Natural Health for Women.* Everyone should read my *Macrobiotics for Everyone* to learn more about diet, supplements, and hormones in general. *The best doctor you can have is yourself.* Take responsibility for your health, and cure the very cause of your condition. Be your own doctor.

Testosterone is one of the most important hormones for both men and women, yet proper testosterone supplementation is almost unknown to the medical profession, *especially for women.* Testosterone-related problems include sexual dysfunction, infertility, irritability, depression, poor concentration, decreased sense of wellbeing, prostate disease, various cancers, diabetes, gynecological conditions in women, impaired cognition, loss of stamina, obesity, decreased muscle mass, male gynecomastia (swelling of breast tissue), impaired vasomotor function, osteoporosis, coronary heart problems, and various diseases and conditions we still haven't researched.

All in all, we're talking about not merely longer lifespan, but a better all around *quality of life* by maintaining youthful testosterone levels. 90 percent of men, by the age of fifty, have low testosterone levels, and need supplementation. Most women over forty have lost half their testosterone already. Testosterone really is your friend.

# 1. What is Testosterone?

**M**en and women have exactly the same hormones, only in different amounts. There are three basic androgens (steroids that control the development and maintenance of masculine characteristics), which include testosterone, androstenedione, and DHEA. Testosterone is a steroid hormone which is produced in the testes in men and the ovaries in women. It is needed to form and maintain the male sex organs and promote secondary male sex characteristics in both men and women. It also facilitates muscle growth, as well as bone development and maintenance. Figure 1.1 below represents the chemical composition of testosterone.

$C_{19}H_{28}O_2$

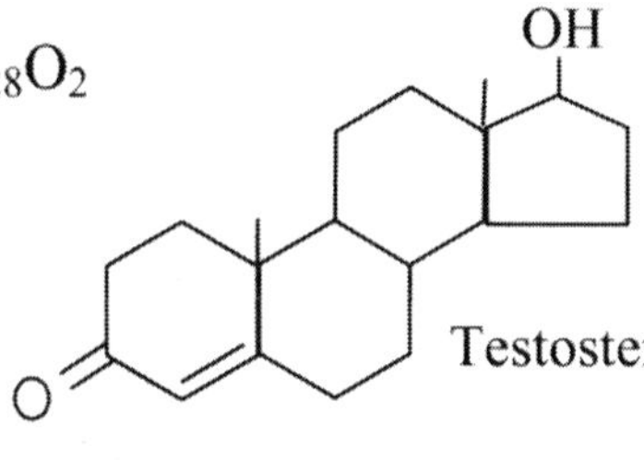

OH

O

Testosterone, CAS 58-22-0

17 beta-hydroxy-4-androsten-3-one     mol. wt. 288.41

**Figure 1.1.** Testosterone Molecule

*Men produce about 6 to 8 milligrams of testosterone per day* in their youth (*Journal of Endocrinal Investigation* v 26, 2003). Women produce about one twentieth of that—approximately 300 micrograms. Women have about one tenth the blood level of testosterone that men have, as men retain it more efficiently.

## TESTOSTERONE IN MEN

Testosterone is the principle male sex hormone. It plays a key role in reproductive function, maintenance of muscle bulk and bone mass, and the growth of body hair. In young boys, the hormone sets in motion the deepening of the voice, body hair growth patterns, and increased muscle strength and mass.

Men produce testosterone in their testicles and adrenal glands, and cannot naturally overproduce this hormone. There is no such condition as "hypergonadism"—excessive levels of testosterone—in men. The only way men can have too much testosterone is by taking some type of supplement. Even then, the male body will only allow so much blood testosterone, and then turns any excess into estradiol and estrone. This is done by "aromatization," using the enzyme aromatase. Androstenedione and androstenediol levels generally parallel those of testosterone. DHEA generally falls in both men and women as they age. Hyper levels are not common, but do exist.

## TESTOSTERONE IN WOMEN

Although testosterone is thought of as a "male hormone," it also plays an important role in women. It is important for bone strength, lean muscle mass and strength, and a general sense of wellbeing. Women produce testosterone basically with their ovaries and adrenal glands. Prior to menopause they can, and sometimes do, overproduce it, and suffer from the masculinizing effects of "androgenicity." After menopause, testosterone levels generally fall, but excess amounts are still possible even after a hysterectomy. Improper female testosterone levels can cause serious problems in women, such as various cancers, obesity, polycystic ovaries, osteoporosis, diabetes, and cardiovascular disease.

Androstenedione levels can also be too high, and excessive DHEA levels in women can contribute to androgenicity as well. One third of American women are unnecessarily castrated by the medical profession, and have their uterus removed. *The ovaries always atrophy and die after a hysterectomy,* despite the constant denials by the doctors. Let's repeat that— *the ovaries always die after a hysterectomy.* This means one third of women over the age of forty have their hormone levels seriously disrupted, and their entire endocrine (hormone) system is completely disrupted.

## TESTING LEVELS OF TESTOSTERONE

Doctors almost never test testosterone, or any other hormone levels. They do not know how to properly test them, or what ideal levels are. Further, they do not know how to raise testosterone levels safely, effectively, and naturally. You simply *cannot* look to the medical profession for help here. You are better off testing your own hormone levels without a doctor. Use saliva or blood testing kits, or Internet blood testing. Google "online blood testing labs." You can order any needed prescription hormones (such as testosterone, HGH, T3, and T4) legally from foreign pharmacies on the Internet.

## CONCLUSION

Testosterone is an important hormone for both men and women, especially for those over forty years old. Most of the research on testosterone is done on males, since it is erroneously considered "the male hormone." Just because men have ten times the blood levels of testosterone does not make it any less important in women. The published international, clinical literature overwhelmingly proves how vital youthful testosterone levels are to both men and women for countless reasons.

Throughout this book, it will be repeated over and over that *all of your hormones work together harmoniously as a team*. Your basic hormones must be in balance for them to be as effective as possible. Please read Chapter 17, "Your Other Hormones," carefully.

# 2. Testosterone Precursors

There are a variety of over-the-counter testosterone precursors that are said to be designed to directly or indirectly increase the amount of testosterone found in the blood. These include muira puama, homeopathic testosterone, Lepidium root, Tribulus terrestis, zinc formulations, tongkat ali (*Longifolium*), various herbal combinations, and other such concoctions. *Science has shown all of them to be useless.* Studies prove *none* of these have any value whatsoever, and are simply well advertised scams. The only precursors that have any possible potential value are prescription drugs such as suicide aromatase inhibitor androstenedione analogs, HCG, aspartic acid, and various steroids like nandrolone.

## ANDROSTENEDIONE AND ANDROSTENEDIOL

Androstenedione and androstenediol are the precursors of male and female sex hormones. They are produced in the adrenal glands and gonads. Their chemical compositions can be observed in Figure 2.1 on the following page. If you merely add a hydrogen atom to androstenedione, you get testosterone. If you remove a hydrogen atom from androstenediol, you also get testosterone. Both of these are the direct biological precursors in all mammals.

Androstenedione and androstenediol are effective precursors to raise testosterone. They were over-the-counter supplements for years. Unfortunately, they are both illegal now, and unavailable even by prescription. Possession of these became a serious felony under the Steroid Hormone Act.

5

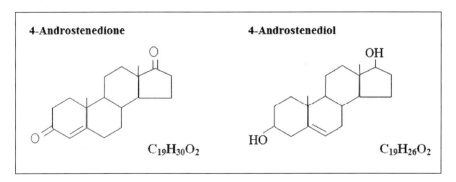

**Figure 2.1.** Chemical Compositions of 4-Androstenedione
and 4-Androstenediol

## ANDROGEN RESISTANCE

An unknown number of men and women are naturally androgen resistant, or become androgen resistant. They cannot use testosterone, DHEA, any form of androstenedione, aspartic acid, HCG, or steroids. Some can't even use pregnenolone, the "grandmother hormone." Pregnenolone metabolizes into 17-hydroxy pregnenolone, and then to DHEA. DHEA then turns into both androtenedione and androstenediol, which then make testosterone. Some people become androgen resistant after using any of these hormones for a period of time. This situation occurs in both sexes.

Using any of these hormones (even aspartic acid) simply turns into estradiol and estrone. It does not matter how the hormone is administered, as this is a biological metabolic problem. How can you tell? Take your androgen for thirty days, and then saliva test for testosterone and estrone and estradiol. If your testosterone did not go up, but your estrone and/or your estradiol did, then you are androgen resistant.

There is zero international research on androgen resistance. With all the testosterone and other hormone studies, there is simply no information at all about people who cannot take androgens. What are they to do? There is no answer, and will not be one for a long time. Cycling androgens does not help. HCG and pregnenolone are not even androgens. Aspartic acid isn't even a hormone. Strangely enough, *there is no discussion of androgen resistance in the international literature.* Using substances like human chorionic gonadatropin (HCG) is just not advised, anyway.

Only about 10 percent of pregnenolone or DHEA is actually absorbed into your blood when taken orally. 7-keto DHEA is an overpriced scam. Overdoses of DHEA (over 25 mg for men and 12.5 mg for women) will spill over into testosterone in men and women who are not androgen resistant. Overdoses of pregnenolone (over 50 mg in men and 25 mg in women) will also spill over into testosterone in such men. In androgen resistant people, these just spill over into estrogen. This situation shows the importance of testing your blood or saliva levels when you are using supplemental hormones. If a person notices water retention, gynecomastia, abdominal adiposity, or any other classic symptoms of estrogen dominance, they should immediately do an inexpensive saliva test of their testosterone, estrone, and estradiol.

## AROMATIZATION

As stated in Chapter 1, men produce testosterone in their testicles and adrenal glands, and cannot naturally overproduce it. The only way men can have an excess level of testosterone is by taking some type of testosterone supplement. Even then, the male body will only allow so much blood testosterone, and then turns any excess into estradiol and estrone through the process of aromatization.

Hyper-aromatization is due to excessive production of the enzyme aromatase, which turns androgens into estrogens. There are anti-aromatase drugs like Arimidex, but they are so toxic they cannot possibly be used. The side effects are terrible. There are no effective natural anti-aromatase supplements, despite the claims. Such things as chrysin and apigenin just don't work well at all. Even the suicide aromatase inhibitors like androstatrienedione (ATD) reverse on you after a while and raise estrogens.

## HOW TO OBTAIN TESTOSTERONE

Always remember that men only make about 6 to 8 mg of testosterone a day in their youth. A proper ballpark dose is 3 mg of natural unsalted testosterone, or 4 mg of enanthate or other salt, in their blood. People with youthful levels should not take any at all. Women only produce about one twentieth of that, or about 300 mcg, and only need about 150 mcg in their blood (150 mcg natural unsalted testosterone or 200 mg enanthate or other salt). 80 percent of transdermal testosterone is wasted, since only about 20 percent is absorbed. This is obviously not the ideal. 99 percent of sublingual testosterone is absorbed.

Transbuccal (in the mouth) troches and transdermal patches are very expensive. Nasal sprays and DMSO solutions are not allowed by law. There are foreign Internet pharmacies sites selling liquid, injectable, natural testosterone in water, or salts in vegetable oil. In the United States, it is perfectly legal for you under United States Code 21, Section 331 to order (use registered mail) or personally import drugs from foreign countries for your own personal use up to fifty dosage units. Just Google the phrase "buy testosterone online" and you'll find numerous sites.

## CONCLUSION

Medical doctors, including endocrinologists, life extension specialists, and holistic practitioners, almost never use sublingual testosterone salts, and uncommonly use transdermal creams. They cannot by law use transdermal DMSO solutions or even nasal sprays. Taken orally, the conversion is a mere 10 percent, which means you get 90 percent unwanted metabolites. Not a good choice at all in the real world. Steroids, even nandrolone (which is natural) and boldenone, are poor choices for a lot of reasons. The only safe, practical, and effective way to raise testosterone is to use real prescription testosterone sublingually, transdermally, or in DMSO.

# 3. What is Your Testosterone Level?

**N**atural hormones are a vital cornerstone of our health, but are also very powerful and cannot be used casually. Hormone imbalance, whether it is a deficiency or an excess, causes chronic symptoms and disorders, and an increase in the risk of disease. Thankfully, balancing your hormones can be achieved easily and inexpensively.

Before using any hormone, you must test your levels to see if you are deficient in anything and need supplementation. Hormone level testing will enable you to monitor your hormones, to make sure they all remain balanced and within an optimal, healthy range. Ideally, you want to know the levels of all your basic hormones. Women also need to check their estriol levels. You will never enjoy the best of health until your basic hormones are at youthful amounts.

## BLOOD AND SALIVA ANALYSIS

There are three ways to test your free biological testosterone level. One, you can get your blood tested by a physician. This is expensive, requires office visits, expensive tests, and is completely unnecessary. Two, you now see blood tests offered inexpensively, on the Internet, without a doctor. Three, you can simply test your own level by using a saliva testing kit. These saliva kits are readily available on the Internet, and will be in the chain drug stores and pharmacies one day. You can pay as little as $35 per hormone to test your testosterone, DHEA, melatonin, estradiol, estrone, and estriol.

9

You also have to use blood analysis for T3, T4, progesterone, insulin, and growth hormone. Women can check their prolactin, LH and FSH levels as well, but this is very optional. You simply send in a saliva sample to be analyzed by RIA (radioimmunoassay). You don't need a doctor, but California, Maryland, Rhode Island, and New York ban people from doing this! The medical profession does not want you to have any freedom whatsoever for self-diagnosis or self-medication. If you live in these states, simply have your results sent to a friend or relative in another state to get around these restrictive laws. Google "online blood testing" and go to sites like www.walkinlab.com.

Measuring free, bioavailable, unbound hormones using saliva or blood spots has been known to scientists for over three decades now. In the last few years, it has finally been brought to the consumer. This is one of the greatest technological breakthroughs in medicine, but is still relatively unknown. The validity, and reliability, of saliva and blood spot hormone testing has been proven for decades. Overall, the results are very consistent. You just have to use a reliable, well established testing facility with a good reputation.

Surprisingly, you usually cannot compare levels from one lab to another, except by general terms such as "low normal" or "below range." Whether you test your blood or saliva, you cannot take those numbers and compare them to another lab, unless they have the exact same range. There is simply no way to convert saliva results to blood results, or vice versa. Add high and low range and divide by two for a midrange value. There are no universal ranges as there are with cholesterol, insulin, and blood glucose.

## URINE TESTS

Some practitioners erroneously advocate urine testing to determine your hormone or mineral levels. Urine is a waste product, and tells us what the body is excreting and doesn't want. The same holds true with toxic elements like mercury or cadmium, which require actual blood diagnosis. A study from the Chinese University, in Hong Kong, (*Clinica Chimica Acta*, v 236, 1995) proves this. Healthy, normal men were tested for their testosterone and estradiol levels, both by blood and urine. They did not find a good correlation at all between these. They stated, "Serum estradiol showed no significant correlation." As men age, their blood and saliva estradiol and estrone (but not their estriol) levels go up dramatically, but not their excretion of these estrogens.

## WHAT IS A HEALTHY LEVEL OF TESTOSTERONE?

Testosterone is a very powerful hormone, and you absolutely cannot use it unless you first prove you have low normal levels, or below normal levels. Medical doctors generally tell you that you're fine if your hormone levels are "in range" for your age. *This is not true at all.* The ideal is *youthful* levels you had at about age thirty. *Youthful levels are the key to good health and life extension.* If you are seventy, you certainly don't want the same levels as all the other seventy year olds, do you? It is important to realize that men and women who are vegetarians or macrobiotics, and do not eat red meat and dairy foods, have lower levels of sex hormones than carnivores. You can see by the following three Figures below and on the next page that both men and women generally have lower testosterone levels as they age.

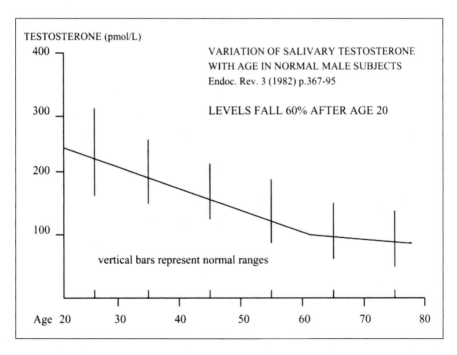

**Figure 3.1.** Male Salivary Testosterone Measurements

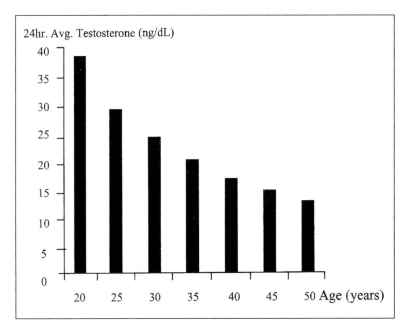

**Figure 3.2.** Testosterone Levels in Premenopausal Women

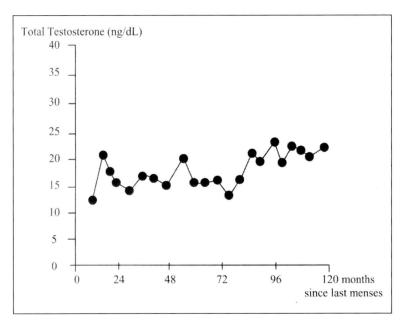

**Figure 3.3.** Testosterone Levels in Postmenopausal Women

## CONCLUSION

When doctors measure your serum or plasma blood levels, they usually test your total testosterone, your bound testosterone, and sometimes your free testosterone. Then they calculate a total-to-free ratio, as if that has some important, esoteric meaning. If you have your sex hormones tested, *you only want your free, unbound, biologically available levels tested.* Giving patients tests that they don't need is simply a fine way for doctors to make money. About 98 percent of testosterone is bound to SHBG (sex hormone binding globulin) and albumin, and is biologically unavailable. Testing your bound and total testosterone levels tells you almost nothing, and is a waste of time and money. Just test your *free, unbound* levels of sex hormones.

# 4. How to Use Testosterone

In the previous chapters, we discussed the symptoms commonly experienced by those with low testosterone. How can you increase your testosterone levels safely? Nasal sprays are illegal for no good reason. DMSO is a solvent that transfers drugs safely and effectively through the skin, but DMSO transdermal solutions are also not approved by the FDA. Skin and buccal patches work, but are very overpriced. Oral capsules are only 3 percent absorbed—the other 97 percent produces harmful metabolites. Surgically implanted pellets are prima facie insanity.

Basically, the only legally available ways to use testosterone are dangerous, unnecessary injections, oral overdoses, surgically implanted pellets, sublingual (under the tongue) tablets or drops, buccal (between the cheek and gum) patches, or transdermal gels or creams. All these forms require a doctor visit, prescription, blood testing, and an extortionate pharmacy price. You'll go broke doing it this way. Doctors and pharmacists will charge you $100 for $1 worth of testosterone powder. Fortunately, you can order your own legally on the Internet from foreign pharmacies without a prescription. You can then make your own sublingual drops in vegetable oil, or transdermal drops in DMSO. Both have about 99 percent absorption.

## SUBLINGUAL DROPS

Sublingual (under the tongue) drops or tablets work well, but pharmacists charge extortionate prices. You can, however, make up your own sublingual drops or DMSO solution. This will cost men less than $3 a month and women less than $1 a month. Men can buy a 10 ml X 250 (2,500 mg) oil suspension of testosterone enanthate. This is 75 percent testosterone and 25 percent enanthate. Simply add 10 ml (325 drops) of vegetable oil (e.g. corn or safflower) for sublingual drops. Add 10 ml (325 drops) of 99 percent DMSO (4 mg per drop) and mix for a transdermal solution. Use a 5 ml graduated plastic medicine dropper for babies to measure this. This yields a twenty-one month supply of either, and would give men 3 mg per day (4 mg testosterone enanthate) of actual testosterone in their blood with about a 99 percent penetration. Women can buy a 1 ml X 100 mg (100 mg) bottle of testosterone enanthate. Add 15 ml (468 drops) of vegetable oil for sublingual drops, or 15 ml (468 drops) of 99 percent DMSO for a transdermal solution. This will deliver 150 mcg (200 mcg) of testosterone enanthate, equal to 500 drops, or almost a seventeen month supply.

## CREAMS AND GELS

Weak, overpriced, one percent natural testosterone gels have appeared in the chain pharmacies. You do not want to use them, as they are 1) too weak (e.g. 1.0 percent) for men, 2) too strong for women, and 3) too expensive for anyone. A compounding pharmacist requires a prescription, and will severely overcharge you for a cream or gel. Never forget you will pay them $50 to $100 for $1 worth of testosterone. Men can get a prescription for 100 grams of a 3 percent cream or gel for under $100. Women can get a prescription for 100 grams of a 0.3 percent cream or gel, and should pay less than $50, even though this is only one tenth of what a man would need, and should cost about $10 in an ideal world. These prices are simply extortionate.

Buy your own creams and gels on the Internet legally through foreign pharmacies. Under federal law United States Code 21, Section 331, you can import prescription drugs for your own personal use (50 dosage units) without a prescription. Sublingual tablets (not to be confused with oral testosterone), natural testosterone, and various salts like enanthate are offered. Also, avoid the various steroids that you may see listed online.

How much transdermal creams or gels should you use? If a man uses a half gram a day, a 100 gram tube (3 percent) will last about six months. This will put 15 mg on the skin, and about 3 mg (20 percent) in the blood. A woman can use a quarter gram of a 0.3 percent cream. This will last over a year. This puts 750 mcg on her skin and about 150 mcg in her blood (20 percent). These are good benchmarks to start with.

Since you probably don't have a chemist's scale in your house, how do you know what a quarter or half gram is? A level quarter teaspoon of most creams or gels (or plain water or oil) weighs about one gram. A half of a quarter teaspoon (one eighth) is a half gram. A fourth of a quarter teaspoon (one sixteenth) is a quarter gram. Be clear that a half gram is about one eighth of a teaspoon, or eight daily doses per teaspoon. A quarter gram is about one sixteenth of a teaspoon, or sixteen daily doses per teaspoon.

## KEEPING TRACK OF YOUR HORMONE LEVELS

It will be repeated over and over in this book that natural hormones are a vital cornerstone of our health, but are very powerful, and cannot be used casually. Before using any hormone, you must test your levels to see if you are deficient and need supplementation. If you have an excessive level, only diet and lifestyle will normalize it.

*Only a total program of diet and lifestyle will lower hyper levels of hormones.* Do not take toxic prescription drugs to lower your hormones, as the side effects will outweigh the benefits. If you find you are supplementing a low hormone, you must test after, say, ninety days. Go twenty-four hours without taking it, and then test yourself about 9:00 AM each time. Only monitoring your free blood or saliva level will tell you if the dose you are taking is the correct one for your individual and unique biological makeup. Further, after taking any hormone and finding the correct dose, you must monitor your hormone levels at least once a year, since your body will be changing as you age. You cannot assume that the dose you are taking will have the same exact effect year after year.

If you are over the age of fifty, you might just assume you are low in testosterone, DHEA, pregnenolone, melatonin, growth hormone, and other such hormones. This is not necessarily true. Even if it was true, you wouldn't know just how low you were in each of these. The scientific way to use natural hormones is to 1) test your natural level to see if you need supplementation, 2) take a reasonable dose for thirty to sixty days, and then test your level again, and 3) monitor your level at least once a year. If you cause excessive levels by over-supplementing, you will have a metabolic imbalance just as serious as with deficient levels. Always remember you are looking for the *youthful* level you enjoyed at about the age of thirty. Hyper levels are pathological levels, and cause serious harm in various ways.

## ANDROGEN RESISTANCE

We should again mention "androgen resistance." This was discussed in detail in Chapter 2, "Testosterone Precursors." Some men and women are naturally androgen resistant, and turn the androgens testosterone, DHEA, steroids (like nandrolone and boldenone), and androstenedione into estradiol and estrone. They can also turn anti-aromatase drugs, omega-3 fatty acids, HCG, DIM, pregnenolone, various amino acids (e.g. carnosine, any carnitine) and other such substances into estrogens as well.

The symptoms of androgen resistance include weight gain, bloating, gynecomastia, and excessive hunger. Some people are born with it, while others develop the problem over time. Those suffering from androgen resistance cannot use any of the types of testosterone mentioned above. Science does not even recognize androgen resistance. There may be no answer to this for decades. Aromatase was only discovered recently, and we cannot even draw the molecule.

## CONCLUSION

Imbalances of testosterone can play a key role in the development of even more serious diseases. Low levels are clearly correlated to a long list of illnesses, including obesity, diabetes, osteoporosis, heart and artery disease, and various cancers. It is only in the last few years that scientists have started to use natural sublingual and transdermal testosterone, rather than ineffective and dangerous oral and injected forms. In the next chapter, we'll look at various published studies showing both the right and wrong ways to use it.

# 5. The Natural Practice

This is going to be a very well-cited scientific chapter. We're going to look at what doctors are doing wrong when it comes to supplemental testosterone and other hormones. We'll learn why oral and injected forms of testosterone are the wrong means of obtaining it. We'll see that low doses administered transdermally, sublingually, or in DMSO, are the most practical, safest, most effective, and least expensive ways to use this important hormone.

Transdermal patches and transbuccal troches (lozenges) technically do work, but are very overpriced promotions of the pharmaceutical corporations. Selling $100 worth of patches, or troches, with $1 worth of actual hormone is outright pharmaceutical extortion. Subcutaneously implanted time release pellets are effective, but are very expensive and have to be implanted surgically. Even the new prescription one percent gels, sold in the chain pharmacies, are weak and very overpriced. Also, the doctors recommend far too much of these gels be applied. The compounding pharmacists will vastly overcharge you for a transdermal cream or sublingual drops. These only contain a mere dollar's worth (in the case of women, about 10 cents' worth) of actual testosterone. DMSO delivery and nasal sprays are not allowed by law, so they can't be studied in clinics. If you take any form of testosterone orally, it will basically be broken down as it passes through the liver. If you take large amounts (i.e. 120 mg for men) orally of an ester salt like cyprionate or undecanoate, only a very small percent of it will be absorbed. Lots of unwanted toxic metabolites will be produced, with serious side effects resulting.

Let's look at some studies on the various delivery systems to see what works, what doesn't work, and why. You'll see why you should test your own levels and buy your own hormones online.

## ORAL MEDICATIONS

At the University of Munster in 2002 (*European Journal of Endocrinology*
v 146), hypogonadal (testosterone deficient) men were given 120 mg a
day of oral medication. This shows how poorly oral testosterone salts
are absorbed to give them literally 3,000 percent (thirty times) what
they need. *Men only make 6 to 8 mg a day in their youth, and need only
about 3 to 4 mg as a daily supplement.* Of course their estrogen levels went
off the scale. Even though these men were given the wrong type of
testosterone in the wrong way, they still got some benefits—albeit with
negative side effects. If they had used proper transdermal or sublingual
forms, they would have gotten better benefits, and no side effects from
estrogen excess.

In 1996, at the famous UCLA in Torrance, (*Journal of Clinical Endocrinology & Metabolism* v 81) hypogonadal men, aged nineteen to sixty,
were given sublingual testosterone. The poor men were given 15 mg
doses (four times what they needed). This made their testosterone go
up about 500 percent, *and their estradiol almost 400 percent.* Using the
sublingual route is very effective, but the wrong dose was used. The
men still got some short term benefits, including increased lean muscle
mass (but not less body fat), more strength, better bone metabolism,
and better blood parameters. If they had given these men proper 4 mg
doses, there would have been no side effects. The real value of this
hard-to-find study is that the sublingual route is the most effective natural legal means we have in regards to actual absorption. Salts, such
as enanthate, are used because they are tasteless. Free-base unsalted
testosterone tastes terrible.

## INJECTABLE SALTS

Injections of ester salts like propionate or enanthate are absolutely the
worst possible means of delivery and pose a danger to your health.
The problem here is that you get a huge rise in testosterone way over
the normal range. This quickly falls until you are back to your subnor-
mal levels by the next injection—a hormonal roller coaster. Even worse,
your estrone and estradiol levels rise to dangerous and toxic levels.
Injections are completely unnecessary, cause extreme highs and lows,
and raise estrogens.

# PATCHES

Some very good work was done by SmithKline Beecham pharmaceuticals in 1996 (*Journal of Clinical Pharmacology* v 36). They used expensive patch "delivery systems." A year's worth of patches only contain about $12 worth of testosterone, but they charge over $1,200 a year! The obscene profit margin is quite obvious. Hypogonadal men aged thirty-five to fifty-six were used. Only about 20 percent of the Androderm® patches actually go into the blood. The 2.5 mg (contains 12.5 mg) delivered dose barely raised their levels to low normal. The 5 mg (contains 25 mg) dose brought up the levels by about 50 percent into normal desired range. The 7.5 mg (contains 37.5 mg) put the men unnecessarily into the high normal range with estrogen overload. The point here is that 4 mg should actually enters the bloodstream in men. Women would only need 750 to 1,500 mcg (microgram) patches to deliver about 150 to 300 mcg. Women utilize this more efficiently than men.

SmithKline Beechum did another study in 1998 (*Journal of Clinical Pharmacology* v 38). Here they just used the 5 mg dose (25 mg patch), since it was the most practical and effective. They used the patches on thin skin, such as the back. DHT, estradiol, and estrone did not go up with such normal doses. The only drawback here is the high cost of the patches.

More studies on the Androderm® patches were done at the famous Karolinska Institute in Sweden in 1997 (*Clinical Endocrinology* v 47). The men, aged twenty-one to sixty-five, were given the 5 mg delivered patches. These raised their testosterone immediately to desired youthful levels, without raising estradiol or DHT. The men were first subjected to harmful 200 mg testosterone enanthate injections every three weeks. These produced the usual erratic high and low testosterone extremes, and high estrogen levels. Intra-muscular (IM) injections gave extreme peaks of 42 nmol and extreme lows of only 7 nmol (normal is about 24 nmol). The patches, on the other hand, produced excellent and consistent results. The usual physical and psychological benefits were achieved, including curing gynecomastia (male breast growth), weight loss, increased libido, less depression, and improved mood.

At the well-known Johns Hopkins Center in Baltimore (*JCEM* v 86, 2001), a more professional study was done with seventy references. The transdermal patches were used with excellent results. Hypogonadal men, aged twenty-one to sixty-five, were first given IM injections. This, as usual, resulted in extreme blood testosterone fluctuations way over and way under range. The estradiol and estrone levels rose to dangerous levels as always. However, the men using the patches dramatically improved their vital testosterone-to-estrogen ratios. They found that low testosterone was correlated with higher BMI (body mass index), and higher testosterone with lower BMI. *Low testosterone is very correlated with obesity in men.* There were many of the usual benefits associated with youthful levels. Intelligent, professional studies like this, using proper delivery to produce ideal levels, will change medicine. Doctors like these demonstrate the value of bioidentical hormone replacement.

## CREAMS AND GELS

At UCLA in Torrance (*JCEM* v 85, 2000), the researchers used a one percent natural gel on hypogonadal men aged twenty-six to fifty-nine years old. The mistake here is that they applied 10 grams a day! This is 100 mg of testosterone! This would put about 20 mg into the blood, rather than the 4 mg they need. The doctors claimed a 10 percent delivery, but in actuality, this totaled to a *500 percent overdose!* Levels of DHT and estradiol in the patients' blood rose to dangerous amounts. Estrone levels should have been tested as well.

Applying 20 mg (two grams of gel) and delivering 4 mg (20 percent) into the blood would have given good basic results. The doctors noted that the average male youthful production is only 6 to 7 mg a day. Imagine slathering ten grams of gel (100 mg of testosterone) on your body every day! A 500 percent overdose. If they had done the equivalent with women, they would have used one gram of gel with 10 mg of testosterone (2 mg absorbed rather than about 0.2 mg). That would have been a 1,000 percent overdose. This would have caused severe androgenicity. Women would only need about one tenth of one gram of this gel.

In a third study published in the same journal, the UCLA researchers cut the dose down to 5 grams of gel (50 mg of testosterone). This is still 10 mg in the blood and a 250 percent overdose. They found that men increased lean muscle mass and strength, had better blood parameters, decreased fat mass, improved their mood, enhanced their sexual activity, and generally benefited dramatically from the treatment. *They overlooked the severe rise in estrogens.* They claim their hydroalcoholic gel only delivers less than 12 percent of the contained testosterone. This isn't true, as absorption is 20 percent for creams and gels. The correct dose would have been 2 grams of gel (20 mg of testosterone with 4 mg delivered).

## A COMBINATION OF ALL FOUR DELIVERY SYSTEMS

A revealing study was done at Koln University in Germany in 1999 (*Metabolism Clinics and Experiments* v 48). Here, hypogonadal men were given four different delivery systems: 1) 100 mg oral mesterolone, 2) 160 mg oral undecanoate ester, 3) 250 mg IM-injected enanthate ester every second day, and 4) a 1,200 mg crystalline (SC) subcuteaneous implant. Mesterolone is a dangerous, toxic anabolic steroid, and 25 mg is the normal dose, not 100 mg. Huge oral doses of esters are toxic, and raise estrogen levels. Such dangerous injections of esters every two days have severe side effects. A crystalline implant of 1,200 mg delivers far too much testosterone too quickly. The doctors observed that the men's total cholesterol, LDL, and triglycerides rose, while HDL fell, but at a dangerous price.

Men over forty were studied (*Archives of Internal Medicine* v. 166, 2006) for overall mortality compared to their testosterone level for a period of eight years. Their criteria said only 19 percent were low. Actually, over 80 percent of them were low. *Men with low levels had a stunning 88 percent greater risk of all cause mortality during this time.* This is just for one hormone. Imagine the benefits of balancing all your basic hormones for longevity.

At the University of Sapienza (*Clinical Endocrinology* v 63, 2005), an extensive meta-review was done of other studies. Such meta-reviews are very comprehensive. They found no doubt that testosterone replacement has many powerful benefits, including increased lean muscle mass, lower cholesterol, stronger bones, and other diagnostic measurements.

## CONCLUSION

The extortionate office fees, blood tests, and prescription prices surrounding hormone testing will bankrupt the common person. Finding a doctor who will even write a prescription for transdermal or sublingual testosterone can be very difficult. Doctor visits and blood tests are very expensive. The foreign Internet pharmacies usually don't sell the creams or drops, only testosterone solutions or powders. You can easily make your own, as we discussed earlier. *No hormone should be on prescription status*. All hormones should be freely available over the counter at very low prices. If this was done, testosterone would be available for a few dollars a month.

# 6. General Benefits of Testosterone

This chapter is arduous to write for several reasons. There are countless studies showing the many benefits of maintaining youthful testosterone levels. The amount of published information is simply overwhelming. There is also a lot of overlap with the other chapters as to specific benefits. There is just no way to clearly separate or compartmentalize these various advantages. Patients are continuously led to believe testosterone replacement therapy is "unproven," and may even have "serious side effects." *Any side effects are always due to using the wrong doses in the wrong ways.* This is a review of the general benefits, so there will be some repetition from other chapters.

The great majority of studies regarding the benefits of testosterone supplementation have concerned men. A very few concerned both men and women to some degree. The little research on women and androgens has been concerned mostly with excessive hormones, not supplementing low levels. *We need far more research on women!* As Dr. Bhasin at Drew University says, "[the] last few years in the androgen field can only be described in the words of Charles Dickens, as 'the age of wisdom, [and]…the age of foolishness.'" Women should realize that maintaining normal, youthful testosterone levels will give them the same basic benefits that men get. Women, like men, can test their own levels with saliva kits, or Internet clinic testing without using a doctor. If their testosterone level is too high, they can lower it with better diet and lifestyle. If their level is too low, they can raise it with very low doses of sublingual, DMSO, or transdermal preparations.

Using bioidentical testosterone, and all other basic hormones, in proper ways results in the most dramatic benefits, with no side effects at all. Everyone over the age of forty needs to be routinely tested for *all* their basic hormone levels, and given supplements as needed. Testosterone supplementation results in countless benefits, such as higher muscle mass and strength, cardiovascular health, better mood, clearer mentality and cognition, increased libido and sexual satisfaction, better quality of life in general, longer life, and all the other benefits we've discussed in this book.

It just can't be repeated too often that people of any age who are proven to be hormone deficient receive countless benefits when proper doses are given. There are no side effects whatsoever. There are *never* any side effects to supplementing low hormone levels naturally. *The ideal is the youthful level you enjoyed at about the age of thirty years old.* Even when the wrong doses are given in the wrong ways, there are still some benefits. Since at least 95 percent of the research is done using the wrong doses in the wrong ways, the best means to deal with this chapter is to concentrate on the few studies that used proper doses transdermally and sublingually. Again, scientists cannot use DMSO delivery or nasal sprays in their studies due to the laws prohibiting them.

## SCIENTIFIC FINDINGS

The many published studies on testosterone, and other hormones, are very positive overall. The overconcern with "risks" is always due to using the wrong doses in the wrong ways. Even when the wrong doses and delivery systems are used—which is most all of the time—there are still some short term benefits. The international literature demonstrates that testosterone is vital to bone health, sexual performance, muscle mass, strength, cardiovascular health, cognition and memory, blood sugar metabolism, body mass index and body fat, energy levels, and feelings of wellbeing and depression, among many others.

- A rather amazing study was done over seventy years ago (*JAMA* v 126, 1944) regarding the "male climacteric." This was over seventy years ago! Middle aged men were given injections of testosterone salts (it was all they had at the time), and very dramatic benefits were found in only two weeks! According to the study, "definite improvement in the symptomatology was noted by the end of the second week in all of the cases treated. Sexual potency was restored to normal with these doses (25 mg IM five days a week) in all but two out of twenty-nine cases." This was groundbreaking stuff seven decades ago, and these pioneer researchers are to be congratulated.

- At the University of the Andes (*Archives Andrology* v 41, 1998), Venezuelan men were given transdermal testosterone. They got very good results, as always, especially regarding bone health and osteoporosis: "The benefits conferred by testosterone replacement therapy are substantial, both in the short term for the eradication of symptoms of androgen deficiency, and in the long term for the prevention of osteoporosis." The researchers pointed out that replacement produces "an overall improvement in mood and sense of wellbeing, energy, friendliness, and a decline in anxiety, anger, sadness, nervousness, and irritability." They talk about the importance of testosterone for heart and artery health. Remember that back in 1998, transdermal delivery was really cutting edge technology. Very good work here.

- At the University Studiorum in Italy, (*Journal of Endocrinological Investigation* v 23, 2000), a review was published covering the entire spectrum of benefits, and various delivery systems. The doctors concluded that the natural means of transdermal and buccal (lozenges inside the mouth) systems were most effective. The effects of testosterone for liver, blood lipids, blood disorders, reproductive organs, skin and hair, muscle, immunity, bones, and sexuality were all discussed. The doctors also showed the value of testosterone replacement in such various conditions as obesity, diabetes, and aging in general.

- At the New England Research Institute (*JCEM* v 72, 1991), aging was discussed, with emphasis on testosterone. The researchers brought up a very important point, in that *illness in general is clearly associated with lower testosterone levels*. This is also true as to how fast and how well we age. *Low testosterone equals all cause mortality.* Keeping youthful testosterone levels just keeps us healthier, and adds to our years.

The New England researchers stated, "The lower levels of testosterone in the less healthy men, which were maintained between ages thirty-nine to seventy years, might be causes, effects, or mere correlates of disease." They used the famous Massachusetts Male Aging Study as their basis, which involved 1,709 men. The results would equally apply to women, for whom hyper- or hypo- levels of testosterone all cause mortality. They also found the androgen DHEA to be very important for health and longevity.

■ Dr. Alex Vermeulen, at the University Hospital in Belgium, has done very long term research on testosterone. Unfortunately, his research omits that testosterone is *good* for prostate health, and that low testosterone is a basic *cause* of prostate disease. He claims estrogen falls in men as they age (*JCEM* v 86, 2001), and supplemental estrogen is somehow good for men! He does, however, recognize that testosterone replacement is important, and men lose 60 percent of their free testosterone by the age of seventy. He also realizes that supplementation is called for, even with prostate enlargement. The fact is that literally *90 percent of men at the age of fifty would benefit from supplementation.* Probably half the women over fifty would benefit as well. *Youthful* levels are the ideal, and not average ranges in old age.

■ Lisa Tenover, at Emory University, is also a popular researcher on hormone replacement, and has published many articles on the subject. However, she hasn't included women in her various studies. In her many reviews, she warns about the non-existent "dangers" of androgen replacement. She actually states supplemental testosterone is harmful for the heart and prostate! She doesn't see that *any "risks" are due to using the wrong doses in the wrong ways.* She doesn't even talk about how many women would benefit. Like the mainstream medical world, she doesn't see the value of sublingual delivery as the natural way to supplement hormones like testosterone, progesterone, and estriol.

Nevertheless, she admits there are many benefits to raising testosterone in men and women who are deficient. She feels "4 percent of men in the forty to seventy year age range would be hypogonadal." The facts are that at least 90 percent of men at the age of fifty are hypogonadal, and would benefit greatly by raising their levels of free testosterone. As men age, this becomes 100 percent. She has not recognized that free, not bound, levels are the only meaningful ones. By ignoring the facts, researchers like her are holding back science by actually damning testosterone with very faint praise.

■ Studies have consistently shown great improvements in health generally with testosterone, no matter which doses were used in what ways. For example, hypogonadal men were given patches to place on their scrotums. The scrotum has high alpha reductase activity, and is not a suitable place to apply androgens. Patches, as we have discussed, are very expensive and unnecessary. These men were unusual in that the average age was only thirty-six. They were treated for at least seven years, so the long term effects were documented.

Bone density increased, so their bones got stronger. This proves testosterone is vital to bone and joint health. *All facets of their prostate health were good, including sonogram analysis for actual prostate volume.* This proves 99.9 percent of the medical doctors in the world are wrong about their antiquated ideas on testosterone and prostate health. Their testosterone to estradiol ratio improved greatly, by a factor of more than 100 percent. There were no side effects at all. Finally, the researchers saw that unnatural injections don't work, never did, and never will for many reasons.

■ A massive review of doctors from forty-three United States clinics (*JCEM* v 88, 2003) treated men with both transdermal gel and patches. They got very good results, especially regarding body composition, body fat, sexual function, spontaneous erections, and overall psychology and mood. The improvements in sexual performance were especially noteworthy. The men generally doubled their blood testosterone levels. Of course, there were no side effects, since they were using proper means of delivery and proper dosing. Both the gel and patches are very overpriced for no good reason, except extortionate profits for pharmacists.

■ Some good and heavily documented research came from such well known institutions as Johns Hopkins University and UCLA (*American Journal of Medicine* v 110, 2001, *JCEM* v 82, 1997, and *Drugs and Aging* v 15, 1999). While these studies focus only on men, women will get parallel benefits in every basic way. Oral and injected ester salts, as well as implanted pellets, don't work well, but transdermal patch systems are effective. Monitoring serum levels is emphasized to insure safety and effectiveness. The studies show that testosterone does not cause, nor worsen, prostate cancer.

Body composition, lean muscle mass, physical strength, and body fat are all improved by testosterone therapy. Sexual functioning and genital dysfunction (such as low sperm count and small penis) are improved, but this is no panacea for impotence. The researchers found that many diseases are correlated with low levels of testosterone, such as HIV, diabetes, osteoporosis, and coronary artery conditions. They also discovered "a substantial prevalence of low testosterone levels in men with cancer."

Overall psychology is also improved, especially cognition, mood, depression, sense of wellbeing, and memory. In addition, it was found that "many autoimmune diseases are associated with low testosterone levels." Bones are stronger with youthful testosterone levels. Reversal of hypogonadism is associated with improvement in bone mass, and maintenance of skeletal integrity. Blood parameters such as anemia, hemocrit, and hemoglobin values are improved with supplementary testosterone as well. All in all, we see that as men get older, their testosterone levels fall, which is *clearly correlated with every problem of aging.*

Researchers do point out that women only produce about 150 mcg of testosterone from their ovaries after menopause. *Women with hysterectomies (one third of American women) are generally testosterone deficient.* Studies show they only have about half the levels of normal women. Women may get many other benefits from testosterone supplementation after menopause, but more research is needed. Why aren't these researchers doing this much needed research on women? Why are women ignored? Clinicians are clearly in favor of routine androgen therapy in men as they age. Soon, they are going to be making routine recommendations for women.

■ At Christie Hospital in England, men were given 5 mg of testosterone a day via patches (*Hormone Research* v 56, 2000). The subjects had improved body composition, more lean muscle mass, and less body fat. Their psychology improved overall. Sexual function was much better. Bone density was higher. Cardiovascular health was better. There were sixty references to other studies showing the validity of testosterone supplementation in aging men.

■ At Harbor University in Los Angeles (*JCEM* v 85, 2000), transdermal gel was used, delivering 10 mg a day to men. This may sound low, but it is still too much considering men only produce 6 to 8 mg a day. Delivering 3 to 5 mg in their blood is the needed dose. The researchers concluded that "testosterone gel replacement improved sexual function and mood, increased lean muscle mass and strength, and decreased fat mass in hypogonadal men." There were no side effects compared with the same dose permeation-enhanced patch. This was a long, fifteen page study, with a full forty-five references.

- At Erasme Hospital (*World Journal of Urology* v 20, 2002), a good review of male aging was done, with emphasis on andropause. By 2025, a full 15 percent of the world population will be elderly, and over the age of 65. We can very much improve the lives of people with natural hormone replacement, instead of having a huge group of sickly, dependent citizens. The cost for such illnesses as cardiovascular disease, diabetes, various cancers, and other conditions is just not necessary.

    Aging does not have to mean depression, sleep disorders, dependence, weakness, memory loss, diabetes, lack of cognition, incontinence, impotence, osteoporosis, heart attacks, hypertension, and the endless litany of elderly conditions we suffer from now. Doctors should recommend overall natural hormone therapy as standard practice.

- We can go on all day with the many published international studies. At the University of Munster (*Journal of Endocrinological Investigation* v 26, 2003), they reviewed the many benefits of testosterone replacement. The doctors noted there are no side effects when this is done properly.

- At Gent Hospital in Belgium (*European Urology* v 38, 2000), andropause was discussed. They suggested androgen therapy to be made a routine practice. With all these clinical reviews, why aren't more doctors, especially in America, using these proven means of hormone therapy?

## CONCLUSION

This chapter on general benefits could easily take up the entire book. The scientific literature is full of studies showing many dramatic advantages of giving testosterone to men (and women) who are deficient. We have only chosen a very few of the countless studies. There is no doubt about the need for supplementary testosterone in men and women who are low, regardless of their age. In the last five years, there have finally been more studies on testosterone therapy for women, and this will continue to increase.

We need more studies on transdermal and sublingual preparations, and no more on injected forms or surgical implants. Patches and troches are fine, but the pharmaceutical industry has to stop the extortion. They can sell a one month supply for, say, $10 rather than $100, and still make a good profit. We have to change the courses in medical and pharmacy schools, as well as the seminars doctors and pharmacists attend. Meanwhile, you don't have to wait for the medical profession to catch up. You can test your own hormone levels, buy your own hormones, and monitor yourself every year.

# 7. Cardiovascular Health

The biggest killer of people worldwide, by far, is cardiovascular disease (CHD). There is overwhelming evidence to show that *men with higher testosterone levels have much healthier hearts and circulatory systems,* with longer and better quality of life. We badly need more studies on women. The current research tells us that women with either hyper- or hypo-levels of testosterone suffer from more overall cardiovascular problems.

A most impressive review of eighty-five studies was done at the Danish Center for Clinical Research (*Atherosclerosis* v 125, 1996). Such a lengthy, well cited review leaves no doubt about testosterone being a heart healthy hormone. It was found that "one intervention, eight co-hort, and thirty cross-sectional studies suggest a favorable effect of tes-tosterone and DHEA on CHD in males." The same applies to women. The largest cross-sectional study in 1987 of 2,512 men (*American Jour-nal of Epidemiology* v 126) concluded, "Subjects with prevalent ischemic heart disease were reported to have significantly lower serum testoster-one levels than subjects without IHD." That one sentence says it all.

The University of Sheffield, in England, did more studies in this area than any other institution (*European Heart Journal* v 21, 2000). Here, ninety men were studied. They concluded, "Men with coronary artery heart disease have significantly lower levels of androgens than normal controls, challenging the preconception that physiologically high levels of androgens in men account for their increased relative risk for coro-nary heart artery disease." They further said, "High androgen levels are presumed by many to explain the male predisposition to coronary artery disease. *However, natural androgens inhibit male atherosclerosis.*"

Further, "There is also increasing evidence in the literature to show that low levels of androgens are associated with adverse cardiovascular risk factors, including an atherogenic lipid profile, systolic and diastolic hypertension, obesity, insulin resistance, and raised fibrinogen in humans." Free testosterone levels were emphatically emphasized, *"This study shows that there is a positive associate between low serum androgen levels and the presence of coronary artery disease."* This is exemplary science! *Testosterone is heart healthy.*

## SCIENTIFIC FINDINGS ON MEN

Heart disease has been found to be the leading cause of death for men in the United States. In opposition to popular opinion, testosterone may actually help protect men from heart disease. Studies have shown that men with CHD overall exhibit low levels of testosterone, and that these low levels can have a negative impact on quality of life and longevity. The mortality of men suffering from CHD was actually doubled in those with low testosterone levels.

■ At Sheffield (*Circulation* v 102, 2010), some more very smart doctors gave transdermal 5 mg (delivered) testosterone patches to elderly men for three months in a double blind study who suffered from chronic angina (heart inflammation) The free testosterone levels rose from 46 to 73 (59 percent) on the average. Their estrogen levels did not rise.

   "Low dose supplemental testosterone treatment, in men with chronic stable angina, reduces exercise-induced myocardial ischemia (blocked arterial flow)." Now they could exercise freely. Aside from the cardiac benefits, these men improved greatly in general physical functioning, social functioning, mental health, overall vitality, freedom from pain, and general perception of their health.

■ Another review from Sheffield (*Quarterly Journal of Medicine* v 90, 1997) showed that, "Low mean levels of testosterone have been found in populations of hypertensive men. In males, high levels of estrogen and estrone are associated with increased risks of myocardial infarction, angina, and CAD. Estrogens given to male survivors of myocardial infarction lead to an increased re-infarction rate. Giving estrogens to men with prostatic carcinoma is associated with increased mortality from CAD (coronary artery disease)."

It is obvious that testosterone, androstenedione, and DHEA are heart protective, while excess estradiol and estrone cause heart disease. Another Sheffield study (*Heart* v 89, 2003) found, "…administration of low physiologic replacement doses of testosterone, over three months, in men with chronic stable angina significantly improves exercise tolerance and angina threshold."

■ From Imperial College in London (*American Journal of Cardiology* v 83, 1999), men aged thirty-five to seventy-five were given intravenous infusions of 2.3 mg of natural testosterone. All of them were suffering from angina, and the majority were testosterone deficient. The infusions "increased time to onset of exercise-induced myocardial ischemia in men with CAD who have decreased plasma testosterone." This means the supplemental testosterone improved the arterial constrictions during exercise, and allowed more blood flow. They quoted twenty-two other studies showing the general benefits of testosterone supplementation for improved heart and artery health. Another study (*Circulation* v 99, 1999) from the San Raffaele Institute in Italy confirmed these same facts: "Short-term administration of testosterone induces a beneficial effect on exercise-induced myocardial ischemia in men with coronary heart disease." What could be clearer?

■ At the INSERM Clinic using the Telecom study (*JCEM* v 82, 1997), obese men were studied. They found, "Compared to the men with higher testosterone, the men with low testosterone had a significantly higher body mass index, higher waist/hip ratio, higher systolic blood pressure, and higher fasting and two hour plasma insulin." There was an important inverse relationship here; the higher the testosterone level, the lower the insulin level. Hyperinsulemia and insulin resistance, with excessive insulin levels, are epidemic in Western societies. Lowering insulin levels is very beneficial in many ways.

■ At the Hunan University in China (*Hunan Yike Daxue Xuebao* 1998), healthy men were compared to men with coronary heart disease. Their sex hormone levels were related to their blood lipids. The doctors found that the higher the testosterone, the higher the "good" HDL cholesterol, and the lower the triglycerides. They concluded, "The results suggest that the endogenous testosterone in males regulates the blood lipid metabolism, and the male with low plasma testosterone might be led to blood lipid metabolism abnormality, a risk factor of coronary disease." Main youthful testosterone levels help keep blood fats low.

When it comes to cholesterol and blood lipids, the literature on supplemental testosterone seems to be less clear. Some studies on testosterone therapy show better total cholesterol, HDL, LDL, and triglyceride levels, while others show no benefits. The reason is that when the wrong doses are given, in the wrong ways, blood lipids are usually not improved. When transdermal or sublingual testosterone is used, there are always improvements in blood fats.

- At Bielanski Hospital in Poland (*Atherosclerosis* v 121, 1996), men with low testosterone were given 200 mg IM injections of enanthate ester every second week for a year. Total cholesterol fell from an average of 225 to 198 mg, and LDL 139 to 118 mg, with no change in diet. Even giving these men the wrong dose of testosterone in the wrong way resulted in some improvement in their blood lipids. The results of the study indicated that "testosterone replacement therapy in hypogonadal and elderly men may have a beneficial effect on lipid metabolism through decreasing total cholesterol and atherogenic fraction of LDL cholesterol." This is the road to good CHD health.

- Similar results were found at the University of Texas in San Antonio (*JCEM* v 77, 1993). The researchers observed "a less atherogenic lipid and lipoprotein profile with increased testosterone concentrations." This included DHEA as well. At the same university (*JCEM* v 81, 1996), some of the same researchers found that low testosterone levels in men equated clearly with high LDL (bad) levels. They concluded that "men with decreased concentrations of total testosterone and SHBG have an unfavorable composition of LDL." They refer to other studies that found low testosterone is also associated with lower HDL levels and higher triglyceride levels.

- We could go on with dozens and dozens of studies like this. To name two more: At Vrije University in the Netherlands (*Aging Male* v 4, 2001) the evidence clearly showed, "Epidemiological studies show, however, that men with cardiovascular disease have low, rather than high, circulating testosterone." At the University of Bari in Italy, (*Metabolism & Clinical Experiments* v 45, 1997) a very in-depth and complex study was done on multiple cardiovascular factors. They said, "Thus, because of the increase of several prothrombic factors, men with central obesity, particularly those with lower androgenicity, seem to be at greater CHD risk."

## SCIENTIFIC FINDINGS ON WOMEN

Hypertension is the most common medical condition in the world. High blood pressure is even a problem in third world countries. Low testosterone is a major cause of this, as well as other cardiovascular conditions. Fortunately, there are some studies on women for this epidemic, but much more are needed.

- One of the few studies that included women was from University Hospital in Belgium (*Sex Steroids Cardiovascular Systems 1st*, 1996). Women can have excessive testosterone levels, while men cannot. Women who have such hyper levels do suffer from more heart and artery conditions, but *youthful levels in women were correlated with less CHD problems*. They went on to also discuss the beneficial effects of normal testosterone levels on insulin function in both men and women. We need a lot more work like this regarding women.

- Postmenopausal women were studied at the Austria Medical Facility (*Diabetes Care* v 34, 2011) for all-cause mortality. The researchers noted that overly high testosterone levels in women are often correlated with heart and artery disease. They followed these women for eight years. Their findings demonstrate low free testosterone levels are clearly correlated with early mortality. They concluded, "In postmenopausal women referred for coronary angiography, low free testosterone levels are associated with both all-cause and cardiovascular mortality."

- There was another female study (*Journal of the American College of Cardiology* v 56, 2010) in which elderly women with chronic heart failure (CHF) were given supplemental testosterone by patch. They were given very extensive tests, such as ECGs, after six months. The results were very dramatic. They summarized, "Testosterone supplementation improves function capacity, insulin resistance, and muscle strength in women with advanced CHF. Testosterone seems to be an effective and safe therapy for elderly women with CHF." More doctors need to be aware of such findings.

■ Testosterone imbalance unfortunately affects adolescent women as well. At the University St. Orsola Hospital (*JCEM* v 98, 2013), girls sixteen to nineteen years of age were studied. 13 percent had menstrual irregularities, and 16 percent suffered from hyperandrogenism. This means one in seven of these girls had hyper levels of androgens. This is the first time the literature reported that adolescent girls have testosterone imbalance. This is not limited to adult women at all. We need more studies on adolescent females, as they often have hormone imbalances that are not addressed.

## CONCLUSION

As the research presented in this chapter shows, there is no doubt that youthful testosterone levels are heart healthy. We need more studies done on women, but current research, common sense, and logic tell us that women with normal, youthful testosterone levels enjoy the same protective benefits as men. As we do more studies on women, we'll demonstrate this situation. Women must be careful to maintain normal range levels, as excessive androgens are just as harmful as deficient ones. Youthful levels of androgens (including DHEA), for both men and women, are vital to good cardiovascular health and long life.

# 8. Various Diseases and Testosterone

The proper way to cure any disease, illness, or condition is with *natural diet,* proven supplements, hormone balance, fasting, exercise, no prescription drugs, and avoiding bad habits (coffee, alcohol, tobacco, etc.). Total natural lifestyle, in other words. Various conditions have been studied for their relation to testosterone levels. This work is still almost unknown to the medical profession, much less to the general public. It remains hidden in medical journals. We need more research on how testosterone levels affect common illnesses, especially regarding women. As always, *all our hormones work together in harmony as a team.* This endocrine "concert" is vital to every aspect of our health and wellbeing.

Testosterone is only one of our basic hormones that needs to be measured and balanced (see Chapter 17 for more on this). It has a limited effect if your other basic hormones aren't balanced. We need more studies on how testosterone affects various diseases. The ones we have clearly demonstrate just how important our levels are for overall good health. Keep in mind that men can only suffer from low testosterone, while women can suffer from both hypo- and hyper- levels.

The best study of all was "Androgen Therapy in Non-endocrine Illnesses" (*Androgens and Androgen Receptors* 2002) from Vermont University. It was twenty-three pages long, with 132 references, and concentrated on critical illness in general, AIDS, renal failure, and pulmonary disease. Testosterone possesses inherent overall anabolic effects. When a person is proven to be testosterone deficient, they usually will benefit from supplementation. This is excellent, progressive, and well documented work covering a wide range of conditions.

## DISEASE AND TESTOSTERONE LEVELS

Few people are aware of the diseases associated with testosterone deficiency. The medical community should be using natural hormone balance as a pillar of treatment. In essence, testosterone deficiency is a common condition affecting many aging men and women, depleting quality of life and longevity. Here are some brief specific examples of how testosterone imbalance affects various diseases:

- At the University of Padova in Italy, women with liver cirrhosis had low testosterone as compared to healthy controls. Both men and women with lupus (LE) were found to be testosterone deficient at the University of Mississippi. Men with liver cancer had lower testosterone levels, compared to controls, at Harvard Medical School.

- Young men with Klinefelter Syndrome were treated with testosterone at Arhus Hospital in Denmark with remarkable progress for three years. At the famous Karolinska Institute in Sweden, men with rheumatoid arthritis tested much lower in testosterone than healthy men of the same age.

- At Beth Israel Center in Boston, epileptic men had impaired testosterone production and elevated estradiol levels.

- Men and women with stomach and colorectal cancer generally had low testosterone levels when studied at Provincial Hospital in China. At Pochon University in Korea, a group of healthy men had much higher testosterone than a similar group of men suffering from various pathological conditions. Men with gout had low testosterone levels at Donetsk University in Russia. Liver cancer patients had low testosterone at Xi'an Jiaotong University in China.

- The Tromso Study in Norway (*European Journal of Endocrinology* v 149, 2003) studied chronic disease in men. "Men who reported having had a stroke or cancer diagnosis had significantly lower levels of total and free testosterone." They also found the lower the testosterone level the higher the BMI (i.e. low testosterone equals obesity). Women were included in the Tromso Study, but strangely enough, not in this review.

## AIDS

There has been some good work done concerning AIDS in both men and women. The fact that this very devastating and incurable virus can be dramatically benefited by testosterone therapy shows us great promise in other illnesses. AIDS is not curable by natural means, because it is a product of the biowarfare research laboratories. It is a genetically engineered virus unknown in nature. Restoring youthful testosterone levels has yielded rather impressive benefits for people suffering from AIDS. At Massachusetts General Hospital (*Archives of Internal Medicine* v 164), women with AIDS were given testosterone patches with striking results: "We found that giving natural testosterone at levels that are normal for women produces significant improvement for patients with few other treatment options."

Again, at the same hospital (*JCEM* v 83, 1998), more AIDS infected women with proven deficiency were given testosterone patches. Very dramatic improvement was noted, with no other treatment. At Harvard Medical School (*JCEM* v 83, 1998) the same results were found for women, using 150 to 300 mcg daily. At the New York State Psychiatric Institute, men with AIDS responded well to testosterone supplementation. At Drew University, male AIDS patients, aged eighteen to sixty, were given natural transdermal patches with powerful results. At the famous Johns Hopkins University in Baltimore, hypogonadal men with AIDS were given supplemental testosterone. They were found to have "improved sexual thoughts and functioning, more energy, and improved mood." It is clear that overall quality of life improves with such therapy.

## Alzheimer's Disease

Alzheimer's is an epidemic, and we have no understanding as to curing it. Diet and lifestyle help to prevent it. At the University of Texas (*Aging Male* v 6, 2003), men with Alzheimer's were given testosterone injections in a double blind study: "...testosterone could indeed improve cognition, including visual-spatial skills in mild to moderate Alzheimer's disease." You didn't hear that on the six o'clock news. The same results were found at the University of Western Australia (*Medical Hypotheses* v 60, 2003), including women. Other studies correlate low testosterone with Alzheimer's and senility in both sexes.

## Aortic Atherosclerosis

Women were included in studies at Erasmus Medical Center in the Netherlands (*JCEM* v 87, 2002). The famous Rotterdam Study of 1,032 men and women was most comprehensive in many ways: "In conclusion, we found an independent inverse association between levels of testosterone and aortic atherosclerosis in men. In women, positive associations between levels of testosterone and aortic atherosclerosis were largely due to adverse cardiovascular disease risk factors." Here, hypertestosterone levels in women were correlated with CHD conditions. In other words, *youthful testosterone levels are good for women* (and men).

## Diabetes

Diabetes is a growing epidemic in America, especially among children, Latinos, and Africans. *One in three children in the United States will grow up diabetic.* Other blood sugar disorders are just as common, especially metabolic syndrome (pre-diabetes). At New England Research Institutes (*Diabetes Care* v 23, 2000), 1,156 men, aged forty to seventy, were studied for ten years. The researchers concluded, "Our prospective findings are consistent with previous, mainly cross-sectional reports, suggesting that low levels of testosterone play some role in the development of insulin resistance and subsequent Type 2 diabetes." Many other studies verify that diabetic men typically have low testosterone. On the other hand, women with diabetes tend to have hyper levels of testosterone.

## Lung Cancer

Research has shown a link between aging men with cancer and lower levels of testosterone. These levels are lower than those in men without cancer. At the Gujaret Cancer Society in India (*Neoplasma* v 41, 1994), male (why not female, too?) lung cancer patients were studied for a wide range of twelve hormones, and other diagnostic factors. This was a very impressive and comprehensive study. The advanced cancer patients had 32 percent less testosterone, as well as 47 percent less DHEA. They also had 23 percent lower progesterone (it is rare to test men for progesterone) levels, but 17 percent higher estradiol levels. It is rare and groundbreaking research such as this that shows us how hormones affect disease states. We need much more similar research done in this area. Congratulations to these fine doctors.

## Renal Failure

Kidney disease rates rise every year, mostly due to our intake of twice the protein we need. Waste products build up in our blood, making us sickly. Studies have shown that men with renal failure not only have low testosterone, but other hormone imbalances as well. At Affiliated Hospital in China, men with renal failure were studied (*Hubei Yike Daxue Xuebao* v 18, 1997) for their hormone levels. "Testosterone levels in patients with CRF (chronic renal failure) were significantly decreased compared with the controls." Why aren't urologists using testosterone therapy with both male and female patients with kidney disease of all kinds?

## CONCLUSION

Every year, researchers around the world conduct hundreds of studies that show a correlation between various diseases and testosterone imbalance. Regardless of what condition you may or may not have, you want to keep all your basic hormones at youthful levels to maintain a long, healthy life. This is covered in detail in Chapter 17, "Your Other Hormones."

# 9. Osteoporosis and Bone Health

O steoporosis is all too common, and affects far more women than men. In Western societies, about half of women over the age of sixty-five have serious bone loss. About one in six men of the same age also have serious bone loss. *There are no effective medical treatments for this*, despite the constant onslaught of advertising to the contrary. None of the heavily promoted drugs improve bone density, despite the alluring claims.

Ironically, poor Third World countries have far less problems with their bone and joint health. All bone and joint conditions have the same basic causes, and the same basic treatments. Whether we are talking about bone loss, arthritis, or tooth decay, it is basically the same metabolism at work. The same cures apply: diet, supplements, hormones, fasting, no prescription drugs, no bad habits, and exercise. *The only real cures are natural ones*. Finally, we have some good studies on women, and we have included some excellent ones.

Testosterone and DHEA are both vital for bone growth, as are progesterone and estriol. As we age, it is important to maintain youthful levels of all four of these hormones to prevent bone loss in both sexes. There are many published studies showing that androgens in general are vital for bone growth, maintenance, and the prevention of joint inflammation and deterioration.

## SCIENTIFIC STUDIES

There are many published studies showing that androgens in general are vital for bone growth, bone maintenance, and the prevention of joint inflammation and deterioration. This means low levels of testosterone, DHEA, and androstenedione. Over 90 percent of Americans over sixty-five suffer from some form of arthritis. This is completely unnecessary.

■ Pre- and postmenopausal women were studied at Keio University in Japan (*Environmental Health and Preventive Medicine* v 3, 1998). "Testosterone was positively correlated with BMD (bone mineral density)" was their clear conclusion. They also went on to say, "These findings suggest that endogenous androgens may exert positive influences on BMD." In China, women with and without osteoporosis were studied (*Guangdong Yixue* 28, 2007). Clearly, the affected women had lower testosterone levels.

■ Hypogonadal men with osteoporosis, aged thirty-four to seventy-three, were given supplemental testosterone at Freeman Hospital in the United Kingdom (*Bone* v 18, 1996). These men got excellent results in only six months: "All bone markers decreased indicating that treatment suppressed bone turnover." They said further, "Thus, testosterone is a promising treatment for men with idiopathic osteoporosis, acting to suppress bone resorption." The fact that men in their thirties were already suffering from serious bone loss is rather unsettling. The same results would equally apply to women.

■ Young men were tested at the University of Lodz, Poland, for their bone mineral density, as compared to their testosterone level. The conclusion was, "There was a positive correlation between testosterone concentrations and BMD, as well as T-score, both in healthy subjects and in infertile patients. Results of the present study indicate that attention should be paid to testosterone deficiency in the young age in terms of the potential risk of decreased bone mineral density in the advanced age."

■ At the Institute of Endocrinology in Prague, both pre- and postmenopausal healthy and osteoporotic women were studied. Their androgen levels were measured. Clearly, the ones with osteoporosis had low testosterone levels. The doctors said, "A major decline in testosterone may influence the development of female osteoporosis." At Mersin University in Turkey, 178 women were studied: "Free testosterone and DHEA were positively correlated with bone mineral density." At the Universita di Pisa, men were given testosterone replacement, resulting in "a strong correlation between BMD and duration of hormone replacement."

- At Hunan University in China, (*Journal of Environmental Pathology* v 19, 2000) both pre- and postmenopausal healthy women were studied. They concluded, "The bone mineral density of the lumbar spine, hip, and forearm were significantly correlated with estriol and total testosterone, respectively. Therefore different hormones should be considered in hormone replacement therapy." They postulated that a major reason men have stronger bones is due to higher testosterone levels. Note the importance of estriol.

- At Indiana State University (*Journal of Clincal Investigation* v 97, 1996), 231 healthy women were studied for bone loss, which was "significantly associated with lower androgen (testosterone, androstenedione, and DHEA) concentrations in pre-menopausal women, and with lower androgens in peri- and post-menopausal women." Sex steroids are important for the maintenance of skeletal integrity before menopause, and well as afterwards. Doctors discovered that "testosterone, androstenedione, and DHEA all fell dramatically as the women age." They also found that progesterone fell a full 59 percent on the average.

- Researchers at Emory University in Atlanta (*JCEM* v 69, 1989) did a five year study for both pre- and perimenopausal women. Free testosterone correlated positively with bone density, even after controlling for weight. "These data suggest that women who are still menstruating may have relative deficiencies in testosterone, with reduced bone densities as a consequence. We found that free testosterone correlated positively and significantly with bone density. In summary, these data highlight the importance of testosterone in women's skeletal integrity and stress the critical influence of hormonal factors on bone loss."

- At the VA Hospital in St. Louis, (*JCEM* v 81, 1996) both white and black women, aged twenty to ninety, were studied for their bone health. Bone density declined in all women over the age of forty, although black women had slightly stronger bones, mostly due to their having higher testosterone levels. Most were overweight (obesity has one advantage, in that obese people tend to have stronger bones in order to support their excess weight). It was found that testosterone,

DHEA, and vitamin D levels were all very important determinants of bone strength in both races, and all three fell as the women aged.

■ A double blind study at Washington University in St. Louis (*Clinical Endocrinology* v 53, 2000) included elderly men and women, with an average age of seventy-three years. They gave them all DHEA for six months. Their lean muscle increased, their body fat decreased, and their bones got stronger. The Cardiovascular Heart Study involved 5,200 men and women for six years. An article based on this, with forty-five references, (*JCEM* v 96, 2011) found higher testosterone levels in women is associated with greater BMD, lean body mass, and total fat mass.

■ At the Tokyo Geriatric Center in Japan, (*Endocrinology Japan* v 38, 1991) elderly postmenopausal women had many of their hormones measured, along with their BMI (body mass index). The women with the highest levels of DHEA, androstenedione, and testosterone had the strongest bones and the least fractures.

■ A really fine study came from the University of Connecticut (*Journal of Gerontology* 56A, 2001) Here, patches were used on elderly men. "Transdermal testosterone prevented bone loss, decreased body fat, and increased body mass." It is difficult to build bone and cartilage in elderly people, so studies like this are even more impressive. At the Milwaukee VA, the doctors said, "Serum testosterone was the strongest predictor of BMD. In aging men, low levels of testosterone are associated with demineralization of the skeleton. Immobility and sarcopenia (muscle loss) with this osteopenia in elderly men."

■ In nine cooperating American hospitals (*JCEM* 81,1996), men were given sublingual testosterone. In six months, their lean body mass increased, their muscle strength increased, and their bones were stronger. Testosterone is a vital factor in healthy, strong bones as you age. Be sure to balance all your basic hormones.

## CONCLUSION

The osteoporosis epidemic is a recent phenomenon in history, but it can be ended soon. The above studies clearly prove the point. Androgens, especially testosterone and DHEA, are the bone building hormones. Both men and women should keep their testosterone levels youthful as one part of a program of total bone health.

# 10. Testosterone and Your Prostate

**N**early every medical doctor and urologist in the world will tell you that testosterone is bad for your prostate and makes prostate cancer grow. This has become an unquestionable Sacred Dogma for doctors, but is 180 degrees opposed to reality. The fall in testosterone as men age almost exactly parallels the rise in prostatitis, BPH, and prostate cancer.

This insanity began more than eighty years ago, even before Charles Huggins got the idea to use castration as a cure for prostate cancer! This is prima facie insanity. Men with prostate cancer who get chemically castrated get very sickly from lack of testosterone and soon die. The damage from castration is obviously catastrophic, just as castration for women (hysterectomy) is equally catastrophic. This butchery has continued, but now doctor use chemicals ("ablation") to castrate men instead of scalpels.

Figure 10.1 on the next page depicts the average man's estrogen and testosterone levels throughout his life. As you can clearly see, testosterone levels fall as men age, while estrogen levels rise. Testosterone dominance and the testosterone-to-estrogen ratio are reversed. The probability of developing prostate disease increases accordingly. *Remember, common sense tells you that testosterone is your friend, has always been your friend, and will always be your friend.*

Note that during youth, a man's testosterone levels will be higher than his estrogen levels. But after he turns thirty, his testosterone-to-estrogen ratio begins to reverse, and estrogen dominates testosterone; this reversal is very dangerous to men's health.

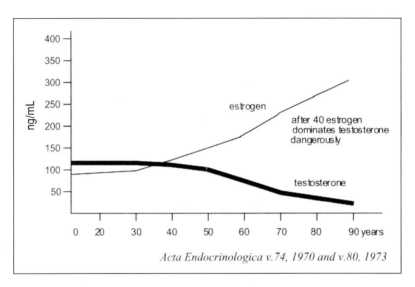

**Figure 10.1.** Average Testosterone and Estrogen Levels Throughout Life

The scientific literature is full of hundreds of studies that prove testosterone is necessary for a healthy prostate and metabolism. When free testosterone levels are low, the prostate receptors must choose dihydrotestosterone (DHT) instead. DHT binding to the prostate is a basic cause of illness. High serum DHT can be harmful to prostate health. Let's take just a few of the published clinical studies to prove that high, youthful levels of the androgens testosterone, androstenedione, and DHEA protect you from prostate illness. Supplementing low testosterone and DHEA levels will help cure your illness. Every month, more such studies are published.

## SCIENTIFIC FINDINGS

There are over 200 published studies in our files from clinics around the world proving beyond any doubt that testosterone helps prevent and cure all forms of prostate disease. In this chapter, there are thirty-one published studies that prove empirically that testosterone is prostate healthy. Every year more such studies are published, yet doctors still chemically castrate men in order to reduce their testosterone levels to zero. Recently, some doctors finally began giving testosterone supplementation to prostate cancer patients with dramatic results.

■ A study on testosterone from Oxford University was published in the *Proceedings of the Royal Society of Medicine* in 1936. Testosterone was only discovered and synthesized in 1935, so it was barely known to doctors, much less available. Ironically, over eighty years ago doctors knew that estrogen was bad for prostate health, and testosterone was good for prostate health. They also were aware of the all-important testosterone-to-estrogen ratio, in which testosterone should control and limit the "female hormone."

■ Another study from Louisiana State University was published in the *Journal of Urology* in 1938. This is eighty years ago! In this case, the doctors understood that testosterone levels fall as men age, and the incidence of prostate disease rises greatly. Doctors gave patients testosterone (from animal testes) with good results. The medical profession inherently knew that "the male hormone" was good for curing BPH, a common malady even then.

■ A progressive, innovative, and pioneering doctor named Richmond Prehn, at the University of Washington (*Cancer Research* v 59, 1999), published a stunning article. He said we should be using androgen supplementation to reduce the growth of prostate cancer! He showed that declining testosterone levels contribute to carcinogenesis, and that supplementing low levels would reduce cancer rates. He referred to earlier studies that verified low testosterone levels in prostate cancer patients resulted in a much worse prognosis. It is doctors like him that are going to lead us into the medical Age of Enlightenment.

■ At the University of Witwaterstrand (*American Journal of Clinical Oncology* v 20, 1997) in South Africa, researchers conducted a study, "Low Serum Testosterone Predicts a Poor Outcome in Meta-static Prostate Cancer." They studied 122 patients, and found that the ones with the highest testosterone levels had the least aggressive tumors, and lived the longest. The patients with the lowest testosterone levels had far more aggressive growths, and died much sooner. The doctors concluded, "Low testosterone seems to result in a more aggressive disease and a poorer prognosis in advanced prostate cancer." This study is very clear.

■ At Hubei Medical University in China (*Hubei Yike Daxue Xuebao* v 19, 1998), doctors studied men with BPH and carcinoma and discovered,

"The results showed that serum testosterone in patients with BPH and prostate cancer antigens (PCA) was lower than that of the healthy control group." Further, "... the ratio of testosterone-to-estradiol is decreased with the rise of the age. The results showed falling testosterone (and rising estrogen) was related to the pathogenesis of BPH and PCA." *It is low testosterone and high estrogen levels that cause prostate problems.*

■ At the University of Vienna (*Journal of Urology* v169, 2003), men with prostate cancer were studied for their serum testosterone levels. The doctors concluded, "Low serum testosterone in men with newly diagnosed prostate cancer is associated with higher tumor microvessel and androgen receptor density (both of these promote malignancies), as well as higher Gleason score, suggesting enhanced malignant potential." In men with low testosterone, the tumors grew faster, the cancer was more aggressive, and the patients died sooner.

■ Doctors at the Memphis Veterans Administration Hospital (*Journal of Urology* v 144, 1989) discovered that elderly veterans fared much better when they had higher testosterone levels. They stated, "Patients with a pretreatment testosterone level of less than 300 ng/100 ml had shorter intervals free of progression than patients with pretreatment testosterone levels of greater than 300 ng/100 ml." The higher their testosterone levels, the longer the men lived; the lower their levels, the sooner they died. This was thirty years ago.

■ In an impressive collective effort between six international clinics (*Cancer Epidemiology Biomarkers* v 6, 1997), scientists used the Norwegian Cancer Registry to study the frozen blood serum and medical records of approximately 28,000 men with an average age of sixty. The scientists found that the healthy men actually had higher testosterone levels than the ones who developed prostate cancer. They concluded low testosterone increases prostate cancer rates. This study is the second largest ever done on testosterone and prostate cancer. *You just can't argue with their conclusions based on 28,000 real men.*

■ The University of Chicago (*JAMA* v 265, 1991) found the exact same results. A separate analysis of serum testosterone levels revealed that the higher the pretreatment serum testosterone level, the greater the survival rate. The higher the testosterone levels were, the longer the men lived, and the better they fared. Doctors should be giving men testosterone therapy, rather than androgen ablation.

- At the University of Utah (*JCEM* v 82, 1997), researchers carried out a rare and unique study of 214 sets of male twins. This is a most effective means of proof. The researchers found that "Prostate volumes correlated inversely with age-adjusted serum testosterone." The higher the testosterone levels, the smaller the men's prostate glands were. This is clear proof that you need youthful testosterone levels for good prostate health.

- At the Petrov Institute in Russia (*International Journal of Urology* v 25, 2002), middle aged men were given testosterone. Their prostates reduced in volume, generally in six months. "These findings suggest that exogenous testosterone in middle-aged and older men with some clinical features of age-related androgen deficiency can retard or reverse prostate growth." Everyone knows that the gradual decrease in male testosterone levels after the age of thirty clearly coincides with the abnormal increase in prostate volumes.

- At the famous Tenovus Institute in Wales (*European Journal of Cancer* v 20, 1984), over 200 prostate cancer patients were studied. Again, doctors found that the men with the lowest testosterone levels had the poorest prognosis, and died the soonest. "Low concentrations of testosterone at the time of diagnosis related to a poor prognosis. Patients who died within one year of diagnosis had the lowest mean levels of this steroid." They went on to repeat, "The results of this study suggest that low testosterone concentrations in men with prostatic carcinoma at the time of initial diagnosis is associated with a poor prognosis. The highest levels of testosterone were found in those patients who subsequently survived the longest." This study was done over thirty years ago.

- Doctors at Baylor University (*Steroids* v 89, 2014) finally came out and said, "Given this physiological concept, many clinical investigators have begun to promote testosterone supplementation therapy as safe in men with prostate cancer."

- At the University of Colorado, a review was published (*Nature Reviews Urology* v 13, 2016). Here, men with prostate cancer were given testosterone. "A recent study review of treating hypogonadal men with prostate cancer with exogenous testosterone found it to be safe." At the University of British Columbia (*Journal of Urology* v 196, 2016), the doctors again found treating prostate cancer with testosterone to be effective. "Testosterone therapy is oncologically safe in men on active surveillance for prostate cancer." At the University of Perugia (*World Journal of Urology* v 31, 2013) the doctors said, "This study supports findings that prostate cancer is associated with low testosterone levels."

- Abraham Morgentaler at Harvard (*Journal of Urology* v 158, 1997) has been the leading proponent of giving prostate cancer patients testosterone therapy. He asserts that "There is not now—nor has there ever been—a scientific basis for the belief that testosterone causes prostate cancer to grow." He went on to say, "The assertion that higher testosterone enhances prostate cancer growth has persisted as a medical myth since 1941, despite all evidence to the contrary." In the same journal eight years later he said, "It may therefore be reasonable to consider testosterone therapy in men with prostate cancer and hypogonadism."

    In *Journal of Urology* (v 163, 2000), doctors found men with low testosterone had far more aggressive cancer: "Low serum free testosterone is a market for more aggressive disease." In the same journal (v 170, 2003), they gave testosterone to men with precancerous prostate lesions (PIN) for one year. Their testosterone went to normal, and they actually improved. Obviously testosterone helps prevent cancer.

    At Beth Israel Hospital (*European Urology* v 50, 2006) Morgentaler said the very same thing. In this journal (v 65, 2014), he said, "The long-held belief that PC risk is related to high serum androgen concentrations can no longer be supported." In the same journal (v 69, 2016), Morgentaler came out and said, *"An important paradigm shift has occurred within the field, in which testosterone therapy may now be regarded as a viable option for men with prostate cancer."* He has published numerous other studies stating this. Morgentaler has been the leading researcher in the world to finally tell the truth.

- In 1978, at the Granada Medical Facility (*Experientia* v 35, 1978), men with benign prostate hypertrophy (BPH) were studied and compared with healthy men. The men with BPH had a 43 percent lower testosterone level than the healthy men. Researchers stated that "the testosterone concentration in the BPH group was significantly lower (43 percent) than that of the healthy control group." They proved it is excess estradiol and estrone that cause prostate disease. This study was published over thirty years ago in a major medical journal.

■ At the Beth Israel Hospital in New York City (*Prostate* v 3, 1982), researchers studied men for thirteen different hormones to determine which ones contributed to the growth of their carcinomas. They found that the average cancer patient had a low testosterone level of about 350 ng/dl, compared to the healthy controls' much higher levels of about 450 ng/dl. In men under sixty-five, the difference was much more dramatic, with levels of 282 ng/dl in cancer patients compared to 434 ng/dl for the healthy controls. This is over 50 percent higher testosterone levels in healthy men without cancer.

■ In 2014, the University of California (*Journal of Sexual Medicine* v 11, 2014) and six other clinics studied the medical records of 149,354 men. This was the largest such study in the world. They ultimately stated that, "testosterone therapy is a viable option in men with a history of prostate cancer." It takes a lot of courage for doctors to make a statement like that. The next year, in the same journal, they published a second study which verified their findings.

■ Thirty years ago at the University of Helsinki (*Prostate* v 4, 1983), hormones were measured in men with BPH and prostate cancer, against healthy controls. The free testosterone levels of the BPH patients averaged only 301 pmol/L, the cancer patients just 249 pmol/L, while the healthy men had a high level of 380 pmol/L. The healthy men had low estradiol levels of only 53.5 pmol/L, while the BPH patients had a stunning 137.4 pmol/L, and the cancer patients 83.7 pmol/L. Furthermore, the healthy men had testosterone-to-estradiol ratios of 7.1:1 (the higher, the better), while the BPH men had 2.2:1, and the cancer patients 3.0:1.

■ Again at Helsinki University, (*Prostate* v 12, 1988) 123 elderly men with prostate cancer were studied for their hormone levels. The researchers concluded, "Low pretreatment testosterone values indicated poorer prognosis." The lower the free testosterone levels, the higher the Gleason score. Lower free testosterone allows the cancer to metastasize, resulting in more tumors. The lower the free testosterone, the sooner the men died. After four years, eighty percent of the men with the higher testosterone levels were still alive, but only 45 percent of the men with the lower testosterone levels were still alive. High testosterone levels win again.

■ At the University of British Columbia, "Testosterone Therapy in Patients with Treated and Untreated Prostate Cancer" (*Journal of Urology* v 196, 2016) was published. Yes, they gave testosterone to prostate cancer patients. The study supported the hypothesis that "testosterone therapy may be oncologically safe in hypogonadal men." Congratulations to these brave doctors. Modern urologists are now able to give their prostate cancer patients testosterone supplements without fear of losing their licenses or being sued.

## CONCLUSION

We could go on with hundreds of more studies on the benefits of testosterone, but these should be enough to show just how strong and comprehensive the evidence behind testosterone really is. Every year, researchers around the world conduct further studies, proving again and again that testosterone is not only beneficial, but also necessary for a healthy prostate. Soon, testosterone supplementation for prostate disease will be standard medical practice.

# 11. Female Sexuality

**W**omen are far more hormonally influenced than men. However, women looking at testosterone as the Magic Answer to their sexual concerns will be disappointed. Yes, it is vital for women to have all their basic hormones in balance as much as possible. Sexuality for women is a multi-factorial and very emotional affair, with far more psychology than biology. "Love to a man is a thing apart; 'tis a woman's whole existence." *Sexuality for women is based on relationship more than anything else.*

Female sexuality is such a complex and multifaceted phenomena, that no amount of hormones could be the single answer to dysfunction. Good sex is a reflection of total physical, mental and emotional health, and not just youthful hormone levels, important as that is. Good relationships equal good sex. Good health equals good sex. We can only deal with biology in this book. Youthful testosterone levels are not even required for sexual desire, as demonstrated by prepubertal girls, postmenopausal women, and those with hysterectomies.

Some women with low testosterone levels have very rewarding sex lives. At least 10 percent of American women are lacking in sexual desire and arousal. 15 percent cannot orgasm at all. *Some studies have found a full 50 percent of women meet the criteria for sexual dysfunction.* Overall, however, women should have youthful testosterone levels for maximum sexual enjoyment. The problem with most all of the published studies is the doctors overdosed the women badly. They just have no idea of the proper doses—about one twentieth of what men need. Yes, men need about 4 mg (4,000 mcg) of a salt sublingually or transdermally in DMSO, while women only need about 200 mcg. This is due to the fact women have much lower blood levels, and metabolize testosterone far more efficiently than men do.

For decades, the effects of testosterone (and DHEA) were studied on men, while women were pretty much ignored. This is changing, and women are slowly being included more frequently in studies. In addition to presenting the studies done on female sexuality and testosterone, we will quote three studies where women were overdosed, only to show how uneducated doctors are about administering this for women.

## SCIENTIFIC FINDINGS

Known factors that affect female sexual satisfaction include age (the biggest factor), hypertension, vitamin D deficiency, excess estradiol and estrone, deficient estriol, birth control pills, obesity, prescription drugs, especially psych medications, alcohol use, smoking, caffeine intake, obesity, recreational drug use, hysterectomy, menopause, insomnia, PMS, PCOS, low thyroid, high cholesterol, diabetes, age, low progesterone, metabolic syndrome, poor diet, high prolactin, high blood sugar, high insulin, menstrual problems, depression, anxiety, CHD issues, and other physical illnesses.

The doctors at the UCLA School of Medicine (*Growth Hormone & IGF Research* v 16 Supp, 2006) put it very well: "Low sexual desire that causes personal distress or hypoactive sexual desire disorder (HSDD) is the most common form of female sexual dysfunction, and androgen insufficiency is one cause of this problem. In addition to a low libido, the clinical construct of the female androgen insufficiency syndrome includes the presence of persistent, unexplained fatigue and decreased sense of wellbeing."

Having said all that, we find that men are not as hormonally affected as women, either physically or psychologically. Many male studies only show maybe a 10 percent improvement in male sexual performance in hypogonadal men who receive testosterone supplements. You will see far more dramatic improvement in women who are testosterone deficient. *Women are simply more hormonally driven than men are.* It is more important for women to have youthful levels of their basic hormones for many reasons, not just sexual satisfaction. Our hormones all work together as a team.

Fortunately, there has been some important research done very recently using proper doses. *Notice when we talk about men, we speak of "performance." When we talk about women, we speak about "satisfaction."*

In a search of the entire published literature of the world, there were far, far more studies on male sexuality than female sexuality. More importantly, for their total health and wellbeing. The real shame here is that medical doctors walk in darkness when it comes to women and all hormones. Most doctors don't even realize how important testosterone is for women's total health. They know even less how to properly administer testosterone to women.

- A placebo-controlled study at McGill University in Canada (*Psychosomatic Medicine* v 47, 1985) looked at women who suffered from surgical menopause after having a hysterectomy (again, *the ovaries always atrophy and die, even if they are not removed*). Most all of these women were testosterone deficient, and responded very dramatically to supplementation. *One third of American women get a hysterectomy about age forty, and lose half their testosterone.*

  "It was clear that exogenous testosterone enhanced the intensity of sexual desire and arousal and frequency of sexual fantasies in hysterectomized and oophorectomized [an oophorectomy is the surgical removal of one or both ovaries] women." The doctors further said, "The major finding that emerged in this study is that on all three measures of sexual motivation, scores increased concomitant with circulating levels of testosterone." The uninformed doctors heavily overdosed these poor women with weekly 200 mg injections. That was 140 times what they needed! Coital frequency and orgasmic frequency were not affected, however. The truth is that 99 percent of hysterectomies are completely unnecessary in the first place. That is another matter well discussed in my book, *Natural Health for Women*.

- Another study at McGill University (*Psychoneuroendocrinology* v 18, 1993) examined the sexual behavior of younger women versus their estradiol, progesterone, and free testosterone levels. They found that "free testosterone was strongly"—notice the word "strongly"—"and positively associated with sexual desire, sexual thought, and anticipation of sexual activity." They also found testosterone was positively related to attention to sexual stimulation. They concluded, "These results are consistent with the hypothesis that testosterone may enhance cognitive aspects of women's sexual behavior." This is a good and well done study. We need many more like this to understand the effects of hormones in general on the sexual behavior of women.

- Further insight on hormones and female sexuality was provided by work at the University of North Carolina (*Demography* v 23, 1986). Here, female adolescents were studied. Levels of testosterone predicted frequency of masturbation (but not frequency of intercourse) for the girls. *It was DHEA, not testosterone, that predicted how sexually experienced they were.* They said, "These (sexual behavior) effects are associated primarily with androgens." Further, "Hormone effects on female sexual motivation are substantial. These effects are also associated with androgens." However, it was *social* pressure that determined female sexual behavior more than anything. Sex is 90 percent psychology and only 10 percent biology, as always.

- At Cedars-Sinai (*Archives of Internal Medicine* v 265, 2005), low-dose patches were again given to surgically menopausal women. Both 150 and 300 mcg patches were used along with placebos. Doctors found that "the testosterone patch increased sexual desire and frequency of satisfying sexual activity after surgical menopause."

- At Amsterdam's Medisch Centrum (*Menopause* v 13, 2006), women of all ages who had a hysterectomy or oophorectomy were given testosterone patches. They had low testosterone and low libido. These women were unfortunately using HRT horse estrogen and progesterone analog therapy Not only did their sexual desire increase, but they experienced more orgasms, were more responsive, their feelings of distress decreased, and their very self-image improved! This was all measured by the well known Profile of Female Sexual Function.

- Remember that sexual dysfunction strongly increases after menopause. Hysterectomies are surgical menopause, and one in three American women will undergo this. At Massachusetts General Hospital (*NEJM* v 343, 2000), women aged thirty-one to fifty-six were give the proper 150 and 300 mcg transdermal testosterone patches after having a hysterectomy or ooophorectomy. The 150 mcg doses gave the best responses.

    This was a double blind study where some of the women got placebo patches. Their sexual function was very impaired from these procedures. Blood tests proved them to be low in both testosterone and DHEA. The patches had very positive effects sexually. They also improved on the Psychological General Wellbeing Index. Imagine if these poor women had all their basic female hormones balanced out! Their overall sexual response not only improved, but also their mood and sense of wellbeing. DHEA is also very important for female sexuality. At Endoceutics (*Menopause* v 16, 2009), sexually dysfunctional women were given one percent intravaginal DHEA. This is poorly absorbed orally, at only about ten percent. Compared with placebo, the Abbreviated Sex Function scale found arousal, orgasm, and lubrication were all very much improved.

■ Another fine study was published in the *NEJM* (v 359, 2008) using the famous Aphrodite Trial. Women at sixty-five clinics around the world participated in this trial. Here, the women aged forty to seventy were given patches which delivered either 150 or 300 mcg of testosterone daily. This is science as it should be. The doctors knew the proper low doses to administer. The Aphrodite Trial was very expensive, very thorough, and great detail was included. This article was titled, "Testosterone for Low Libido in Postmenopausal Women Not Taking Estrogen." Notice that none of the women were on HRT.

■ Community studies show many post-menopausal women continue to be sexually active with their husbands despite a high level of dissatisfaction. They do this to please their partner and maintain domestic harmony. The therapy dramatically improved their level of satisfaction, enjoyment, orgasm, and reduced their feelings of anxiety and distress.

■ At the famous Karolinska Institute in Sweden (*Climacteric* v 5, 2002), the doctors overdosed women forty-five to sixty years old with oral 40 milligram (200 times what they needed sublingually) doses of testosterone undecanoate. Oral testosterone does not work, as only three percent is absorbed. All of the women had hysterectomies and/or oophorectomies. Nevertheless, they found dramatic effects for sexual relations, especially for satisfaction, frequency, and interest in sex. They summarized, "The addition of testosterone undecanoate improved specific aspects of sexual function." If they had used transdermal or sublingually testosterone in proper amounts, they would have done much better.

■ At Utrecht University in the Netherlands (*Archives of General Psychiatry* v 57, 2000), a unique double blind, placebo study was done on women. They were not known to be low in testosterone, and were functioning normally. Surprisingly, these modern doctors used sublingual testosterone. Only one dose was given to study the effects on physiological and subjective sexual arousal. They gave the women testosterone, and then showed them erotic films of couples having intercourse. The authors found "a statistically significant increase in genital responsiveness. Furthermore, on the day of testosterone treatment, there also was a strong and statistically significant association between the increase in genital arousal and subjective reports of genital sensations and sexual lust." Now, this is just with one single dose on normal women not known to have any testosterone deficiency at all. This is *not* to infer that any woman with normal levels should in any way consider raising them to supraphysiological (i.e. excessive) levels. High levels of androgens cause serious conditions in women, just as deficient levels do. The doctors should have never given testosterone to women without testing them first.

■ A very surprising study was done forty years ago at three hospitals in the United Kingdom (*British Journal of Psychiatry* v 132, 1978). Sexually unresponsive women were studied, along with their husbands. They were given personal counseling, since sexuality is far more psychological than physiological. Amazingly enough, they were given sublingual testosterone! The fact that women were given the proper sublingual form, almost four decades ago, is a credit to these researchers. However, they were given huge, toxic 10 mg doses—about fifty times too much—but "only" for ninety days. 200 mcg of enanthate would have been good. The results were nothing less than dramatic, including frequency of orgasm, arousal, erotic feelings, and satisfaction: "Those receiving testosterone did significantly better on a number of behavioral and attitudinal measures." Not only was the women's sexual happiness greatly improved, but their overall psychology as well.

■ Twelve doctors from around the country collaborated (*NEJM* v 343, 2000) to study women after removal of their ovaries. There is very little testosterone produced by the adrenal glands after a hysterectomy or oophorectomy. Sexual functioning in these women is severely impaired. *One third of all American women will suffer unnecessary hysterectomies, at an average age of only forty years.* The women were given

150 to 300 mcg of transdermal testosterone daily, since their rate of production is only about 300 mcg a day.

The doctors stated, "In women who had undergone oophorectomy, transdermal testosterone improves sexual function and psychological wellbeing." They went on to say, "...as reflected by scores on the Brief Index of Sexual Functioning for Women, the dimensions of thoughts—desire, arousal, frequency of sexual activity, pleasure and orgasm—were most affected." While sexual satisfaction was dramatically improved, their general psychology was equally affected: "In regard to psychological status, testosterone replacement had a beneficial effect on well-being and depressed mood." When testosterone is given properly in natural ways, the effects are no less than stunning.

■ National Institutes of Mental Health sponsored a study almost three decades ago (*Archives of Sexual Behavior* v 7, 1978) showing the relationship of testosterone levels in women to sexual satisfaction. Young, healthy married couples were extensively studied with in-depth psychological tests, as well as hormone measurements. Researchers found that "the wives' self-rated gratification scores correlated significantly with their own plasma testosterone levels ... that high baseline testosterone level was significantly related to high self-rated gratification score and the ability to form good interpersonal relationships."

Not only was sexual satisfaction related to testosterone levels, but the very ability to have a better relationship with other people. It was also pointed out that low testosterone was related to anxiety, and high testosterone to freedom from anxiety. This study is over a half century old. Gynecologists and endocrinologists are still not clear about the need for testosterone in women and the proper dosing.

■ Postmenopausal women have a long list of sexual problems, including loss of desire, less activity, fatigue, no sense of wellbeing, and other such issues. At Case Western Reserve University (*Journal of Sexual Medicine* v 4 Supp, 2007), such women were given low-dose transdermal patch testosterone. They responded very well. Overwhelmingly, they found much greater sexual enjoyment after menopause. If all their basic hormones had been balanced out, they would have responded even more.

## HOW MUCH TESTOSTERONE DO WOMEN NEED?

*The proper ballpark dose for women who are proven to be low in free testoster-one is only about 150 mcg (micrograms) in their blood.* Remember that magic number: *150 mcg in their blood.* The best way to do this is with 200 mcg of testosterone enathate (150 mcg of actual testosterone) in vegetable oil administered sublingually. 750 mcg of transdermal (20 percent absorption) natural testosterone cream or gel is also effective.

Unlike men, women can naturally have too much or too little androgens in their system. Androgens basically include testosterone, DHEA, and androstenedione. Women with hyper androgen levels (androgenicity) suffer from many medical conditions, including facial hair, polycystic ovaries, diabetes, obesity, and various forms of cancer. As always, women need to measure their levels of free testosterone, and DHEA or DHEA-S (sulfate).

## CONCLUSION

Female hormones, especially testosterone, influence sexual activity and fulfillment very strongly in all aspects. Research has shown that high or low levels of testosterone can harm a woman's physical health, as well as her emotional wellbeing. The same research has proven that testosterone can work to heighten a woman's sexual drive.

Now the researchers of the world are using proper doses of testosterone with women for their total health and wellbeing. Ladies, you don't need any more studies done. Just test your free testosterone, and supplement it if you are low. If you are too high, just change your diet and lifestyle to lower your level.

# 12. Male Sexuality

The published literature on male sexuality is overwhelming, and much of this concerns erectile dysfunction. Again, we always see "performance" in men, and "satisfaction" in women. Men understandably refuse to discuss this, as it goes to the very core of their feelings of masculinity. The best estimates are that over half of men over seventy-five are simply sexually inactive, *over 40 percent of men over sixty have erectile failure,* and over a quarter of those over forty (*Journal of the American Geriatric Society* v 36, 1988) have some performance issue. *One fourth of men over forty have serious performance issues.* These are high numbers!

Sexual dysfunction in men is very complex, and includes psychology, vascular disorders, hormonal factors, drugs, both prescription and recreational, obesity, alcoholism, and other illnesses such as diabetes and hypertension. The only way to cure a complex condition like this is with a total program of diet and lifestyle, and nothing less than that.

*Good health equals good sex.* Science proves that testosterone and androgens in general are very important to sexual function in men, *but far down the list as to causing impotence. Good relationship equals good sex,* as well. Remember that men should balance their basic twelve hormones, and not just their androgens testosterone and DHEA. Testosterone supplementation alone is not the answer for sexually dysfunctional men. We'll just use studies where sublingual or transdermal forms are used, rather than injected or oral use. Why use those where the doctors don't even know how to administer it properly?

Always remember that *human sexuality is 90 percent psychology, and only 10 percent biology.* Some men cannot function with their wives, but can with another woman. Good relationship is vital here. Some men respond to pornography, but not real women. Some need pornography to function with a real woman. *Good relationship equal good sex!* It is very obvious that happy couples tend to have good sexual relations as a reflection of their relationship. To determine whether this primarily biological or psychology you merely need to know if you get nocturnal erections. Just put a strip of one cent postage stamps around your flaccid penis when going to bed, and see if it is broken in the morning. If it is, your problem is in your mind, not your body. Isn't that elegant in its simplicity? If you can have an erection while sleeping, then it's not physical.

## ERECTILE DYSFUNCTION

A very good study came from the famous Karolinska Institute (*Journal of Urology* v 155, 1996). Hypogonadal men, aged twenty-one to sixty-five, were given transdermal patches that delivered 5 mg a day of natural testosterone (only about 20 percent penetration rate from 25 mg, and very expensive). These doctors are to be given a lot of credit for using transdermal testosterone in normal doses. The patches raised the men's free testosterone levels to youthful levels without raising estrogens or DHT. They gave these men extensive, subjective, and objective tests of various kinds to monitor their improvement.

The doctors concluded, "...nocturnal erections occurred more frequently with longer duration and greater rigidity, and patient assessments of sexual desire and weekly number of erections were higher." They said further, "These findings suggest that androgen replacement therapy has an impact on all aspects of male sexual function, unconscious and conscious." They quoted a number of other studies that found similar results. Research like this will eventually result in routine testosterone testing, and supplementation in normal medical practice. Remember though, while this was a great improvement, it was not a cure-all by any means.

Also note that symptomatic, dangerous, and unnatural chemical band-aids like Viagra®, Levitra®, and Cialis® result in permanent and irreversible impotency. Never use these drugs.

Doctors at the University of Vienna looked at men with erectile dysfunction (ED) for their hormone levels (*Urology* v 53, 1999). They found that low DHEA was a major cause of impotence. Their results suggested that "oral DHEA treatment may be of benefit in the treatment of ED." It becomes obvious that both testosterone and DHEA should be measured and supplemented if necessary in men over forty or younger men with sexual functioning problems. (Androstenedione generally tracks testosterone, and does not need to be supplemented by itself.)

Doctors at Northwestern University did a fine review and meta-analysis of sixteen major studies chosen from seventy-three published ones (*Journal of Urology* v 164, 2000). They stated, "Our meta-analysis of the usefulness of androgen replacement therapy for erectile dysfunction indicates that the response rate for a primary etiology was improved over that for a secondary etiology, transdermal testosterone therapy was more effective than intramuscular or oral treatment..." They found 81 percent of men treated with transdermal forms of testosterone got benefits, but this sounds very, very optimistic. Other studies only got about 10 percent. They pointed out that erectile dysfunction, while too embarrassing to be openly discussed, affects up to 30 million American men. That comes to only 20 percent, though.

At the Association pour l'Etude de la Pathologie in France (*Journal of Urology* v 158, 1997), we find out just how little the medical profession knows about hormones. 1,022 men complaining of erectile dysfunction (ED), were studied, and their testosterone measured. The doctors arbitrarily decided that any man with a level of less than 4 ng/ml was testosterone deficient. This meant that only 9 percent (one in eleven) men over the age of fifty were deemed hypogonadal, and in need of supplementation.

At the University of Modena in Italy (*International Journal of Andrology* v 19, 1996, and *Journal of Andrology* v 18, 1997), two studies were done. In the first, healthy men were divided into four groups according to their testosterone level. Only the lowest group showed problems, as reflected by nocturnal electronic monitoring of their erections: "Group 1 showed significantly impaired night erections when compared with any of the other three groups, but no differences were detected among Groups 2, 3, and 4."

In the second study, healthy subjects were divided into eight groups according to their testosterone level. Their erections during sleep were also monitored electronically. "The groups of subjects with higher testosterone serum levels (400 ng and above) showed almost constantly higher value for the erectile parameters studied than the subjects with serum testosterone less than 99 ng/dL." It must be pointed out that *only the men with the lowest testosterone levels had serious problems* with nocturnal erections. The majority of men simply will not be helped by such therapy.

At the well known Kinsey Institute of Research (*Psychoneuroendocrinology* v 20, 1995), a double blind study with normal and hypogonadal men was done. They were given erotic stimuli, and their erections monitored electronically. Researchers determined, "the number of satisfactory nocturnal penile tumescence (nighttime erections) responses, in terms of both circumference increase and rigidity, were less in the hypogonadal men than the controls. They were significantly increased by androgen replacement, confirming the results of earlier studies." There was good improvement here, but only in the hypogonadal men. Testosterone is only one factor, albeit an important factor, in male sexual performance and ability.

## GENERAL IMPTOENCY

Some important, extensive, and comprehensive work was done at Boston University in 1994 (*Journal of Urology* v 151). This was the famous Massachusetts Male Aging Study (MMAS) on 1,290 average men aged forty to seventy. Fully 10 percent of these men were impotent, and 52 percent suffered from transient or partial impotence. *One in ten men over the age of forty in America cannot function at all sexually!* Over half of them have serious problems with sexual performance.

The older the men were, the more prominent their sexual dysfunction. They found the causative factors to be *age,* heart disease, hypertension, diabetes, prescription medication, anger, depression, high cholesterol, cigarette smoking, and low DHEA levels. Seventeen hormones were measured in these men, but only low DHEA was related to impotence. Testosterone, including free testosterone, was not found to be a factor at all, surprisingly. There are no simple or easy cures for male sexual dysfunction. Alcoholics functioned just fine for some reason, as did obese and arthritic men. Other studies do contradict this. The epidemic of impotence is largely hidden because of the shame these men feel about their condition. This is due to *diet, lifestyle, and psychology* more than anything else.

Folks, the facts of the matter are that at least *90 percent of men at the age of fifty are testosterone deficient,* and could benefit greatly from supplementation. Let's repeat that… *90 percent of men by fifty are testosterone deficient.* Setting the cutoff point at the lowest 9 percent is ridiculous. To use a sickly standard like this makes no sense at all. Low levels found in aging men may be "normal" for their age, but are nevertheless pathological and cause serious problems. The *youthful* levels men enjoyed at about the age of thirty should be the standard. Youthful hormone levels are always the standard. They did find good success with erectile dysfunction, but *only* with the men with the lowest testosterone levels. Again, we see that sex is 90 percent psychology and only 10 percent biology.

## HYPERTENSION AND TRIGYLCERIDES

Hypertension is a major factor in male dysfunction. Many studies have shown high blood pressure to be a major factor here. One study claimed (*Hypertension* v 28, 1996) this is the most important of all biological factors. Hypertensive men have far more erectile dysfunction than normotensives. High blood pressure is basically due to insulin resistance more than anything else, and can easily be cured naturally with diet and lifestyle.

Triglycerides, and possibly cholesterol levels, are also a factor (*Asian Journal of Andrology* v 9, 2007). Men with triglyceride levels over 150 had far more sexual performance problems. Your level should be under 100. High cholesterol comes from eating animal fats in meat, poultry, eggs, and dairy. High triglycerides come from eating sugar of any kind, including fruit juice, honey, and stevia. Other studies have shown high blood glucose levels to be a factor (*Journal of Urology* v 176, 2006), as well as pre-diabetes or Metabolic Syndrome. High blood sugar only comes from eating any kind of simple sugar or using caffeine. Obesity is another factor. One third of Americans are seriously overweight, and sexual dysfunction is just another of the countless problems caused by being overweight. High prolactin levels are a very serious condition in both men (and women). You can get your prolactin tested very inexpensively after you have balanced all your other basic hormones.

## ESTROGEN

High levels of estradiol (E2) and estrone (E1) are a major cause of prostate disease, as well as sexual dysfunction. *Men over fifty generally have higher E1 and E2 levels than their postmenopausal wives.* This is a very bad situation. High E1 and E2 are the internal causes of prostate disease and many other problems in aging men. Only diet and lifestyle will lower hyper estrogen levels. Low fat diet, DIM, flax oil, avoiding alcohol, fiber, and exercise all help lower estrogens. Never use any estrogen lowering drug such as Arimidex®. Estriol (E3) is normally balanced in men of any age, and does not seem to be related to sexual dysfunction. This is called the "good," or safe, estrogen in women.

## CONCLUSION

Impotence and sexual dysfunction in men is a hidden problem they are not willing to admit to or discuss openly. Synthetic chemicals such as Viagra®, Cialis®, and Levitra® are not the answer at all, don't work in most men, and merely deal with the superficial symptom of much deeper problems. We will not discuss the many dozens of studies around the world over the last twenty years that used injections or oral doses of toxic salts. Yes, the patients nearly always got impressive benefits, but only if they were very low in free testosterone.

Fortunately, doctors are slowly waking up to the fact that the correct way to administer non-oral hormones like testosterone (progesterone, estriol, and growth hormone) is transdermally or sublingually. Sexuality is a complex situation and hormones are only one part of this, especially in men. It is your total *lifestyle* that causes—and cures—impotence, not Magic Hormones. Sexual performance in men depends on good relationships more than anything else. Other central factors include *age*, obesity, hypertension, low androgens, blood sugar dysfunction, high blood fats, prostate issues, prescription drugs, and bad habits like smoking and drinking. Good health equals good sex! Good health and good relationship are the road to male sexual ability.

# 13. Women Need Testosterone, Too

It is well known that women are more influenced by their hormones than men are. This is certainly true when it comes to testosterone. Although women only have about one tenth the amount of blood testosterone men do, it is no less important to them. It is estimated that women produce about 300 mcg a day, but retain more of it in their blood than men do. Just because they have a lower level of blood testosterone does not mean it has any less effect on them.

Always remember women can have hypo- or hyper-levels of testosterone. *They must be midrange to be healthy and well.* Medical doctors have no idea how important testosterone is for women, and almost never test them for their levels, much less prescribe supplements for them. The traditional wisdom is that testosterone is "the male hormone," and estrogens the "female hormones." Even if doctors did measure female androgens, they would have no idea of the difference between their bound, total, and free levels. They would have even less of an idea of how to properly administer them to those who are deficient. In the entire scientific world, there are only a handful of published studies—most very recently—on testosterone therapy for women. Only a few of these use proper doses transdermally or sublingually.

One of the best overall studies was from the National Institutes of Health (NIH) in Bethesda, titled "Testosterone Therapy in Women: Myths and Misconceptions" (*Maturitas* v 74, 2013). The authors showed how beneficial testosterone therapy is for women who need it. They exposed ten myths commonly held by most doctors. Testosterone is not a "male hormone." Libido is not the only reason to use it. It does not masculinize women, change the tone of voice, or cause hair loss. It has beneficial effects on the heart. Testosterone doesn't cause liver damage or aggression, and it doesn't increase the incidence of breast or other cancers. The safety for women has been well proven. This is really a stunning piece of work by very enlightened doctors.

Androgen production in women usually falls by 50 percent from the age of twenty to forty (*JCEM* v80, 1995, and v90, 2006). Low testosterone is a major cause of cardiovascular disease. Researchers found that "the plasma levels of DHEA are decreased in patients with CHF in proportion to its severity." Coronary heart disease is the biggest killer of all, far more than cancer or any other disease.

Ladies, you have to be your own doctor here. Test your testosterone and DHEA levels with an inexpensive saliva test. Go to inexpensive online labs that don't require a doctor. Normal pharmacies can't help you. Compounding pharmacies charge extortionate prices, and require a prescription from a doctor. Creams and patches are ridiculously over-priced, sublingual solutions unknown, and DMSO solutions illegal. Buy your own testosterone on the Internet from foreign online pharmacies. A $60 bottle of 10 X 250 (2,500 mg) will last a woman thirty-four years! That's 50 cents a year.

## SCIENTIFIC FINDINGS

Research has shown new evidence that testosterone is an important component in women's health. Over the course of a woman's life, and especially as she ages, testosterone plays a number of key roles in her health. Let's look at some of the very few good studies to show how this hormone can help you if you are deficient. If you have hyper levels, only diet, lifestyle and hormone balance will lower them.

■ The very best study in print was in 2011 (*Maturitas* v 68). Pre- and postmenopausal women were given testosterone implants. The researchers used the Menopause Rating Scale (MRS) to show the benefits of correctly giving pre- and postmenopausal women testosterone supplements. The MRS uses eleven categories of women's health. The questionnaire is very accurate and very effective in diagnosing health issues for women.

The MRS includes:

1. Hot flashes
2. Heart discomfort
3. Sleep problems
4. Depression
5. Irritability
6. Anxiety

7. Exhaustion—physical and mental
8. Sexual dysfunction
9. Bladder problems
10. Vaginal dryness and atrophy
11. Joint and muscle problems

Take a look at Figure 13.1 below. The high bars on the left show the original poor health scores of the women. You can see by the short bars on the right the extremely dramatic results. Researchers concluded that, "Continuous testosterone alone, delivered by subcutaneous implant, was effective for the relief of hormone deficiency symptoms in both pre- and postmenopausal patients. The validated MRS questionnaire proved a valuable tool in the measurement of the beneficial effects of testosterone therapy."

■ *Low testosterone actually causes heart and artery disease and early death* (Diabetes Care v 34, 2011). Researchers have found that, "In

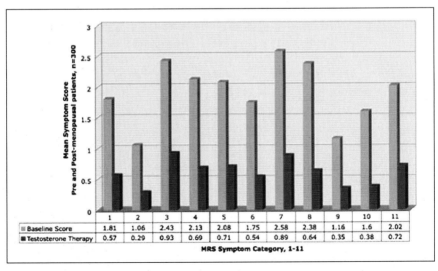

**Figure 13.1.** MRS Scores in Pre- and Postmenopausal Women

postmenopausal women referred for coronary angiography, low free testosterone levels are independently associated with increased all-cause and cardiovascular mortality." DHEA is the second most important androgen. Women with chronic heart failure (CHF) were found to be low in DHEA (JCEM v 85, 2000). There are a good number of studies on the benefits of testosterone for women and CHD.

■ The doctors at the well known Baylor College said oral methyl testosterone "is the most commonly used form of androgen replacement for postmenopausal women" (*International Journal of Fertility* v 41, 1996). Methyl testosterone is the worst possible form of testosterone, and is extremely toxic and dangerous. This should be completely banned for human or animal use. These doctors also claimed testosterone levels in women actually rise with age.

■ The doctors at the famous Vienna Medical University in Austria (*Obstetrics and Gynecology* v 89, 1997) were also misled. The poor women patients were given transdermal testosterone, but they gave the women 40 mg a day! If only 10 percent of this was absorbed (it was in petroleum, which is a very ineffective base for skin penetration), this would mean 4,000 mcg, instead of a reasonable 150 mcg. This is a one month supply every day, or almost *thirty* times what they needed. The women were immediately well over the high range, and started to develop serious side effects. To make things worse, they did not limit the supplementary testosterone to women who had low levels, but gave it to all the women in the study regardless of their level.

■ One of the very few good reviews on women and testosterone was done at the University of Utah in 2002 with an impressive fifty-six references (*International Journal of Fertility* v 47). It was pointed out that women only produce about 300 mcg a day (one third of one milligram), half of this from the ovaries, and half from the adrenals. Contrary to logic, a few women after hysterectomy still have high testosterone levels, even though their ovaries have atrophied (regardless of whether or not they were removed). They discuss "Female Androgen Deficiency Syndrome," or FADS. The researchers found that testosterone falls strongly between the ages of twenty and fifty prior to menopause, but rises slightly after menopause.

- At UCLA in San Diego (*American Journal of Obstetrics and Gynecology* v 118, 1974) thirty years ago, women with endometrial cancer had their ovaries removed. Their testosterone and androstenedione levels fell to less than half immediately after the operation. Their DHEA also fell, but was not measured. No attempt was made to supplement their deficient levels, nor was the concept even addressed! To add insult to injury, they were then injected with synthetic toxic medroxyprogesterone, instead of being given natural transdermal progesterone. Why aren't women with deficient hormone levels, after hysterectomy, routinely given supplemental natural hormones?

## PRE-MENSTRUAL SYNDROME

Most all American women suffer from Pre-Menstrual Syndrome (PMS), and some rather severely. In 1998, at the National Institutes of Health in Maryland (*Biological Psychiatry* v 43), women with PMS and low testosterone levels were compared to healthy controls. PMS is the most common female complaint, and the symptoms can last for up to fifty years after the menses cease. Researchers concluded that "PMS subjects had significantly lower total and free plasma testosterone levels, with a blunting of the normal periovulatory peak, a finding that may be epiphenomenal (related) to age."

This is not to suggest that supplemental testosterone is a "magic cure" for PMS, nor even that all women with PMS are testosterone deficient, but rather it is an important factor that needs to be addressed. PMS is epidemic in Western cultures, but not in Asian or African cultures. Women suffering from PMS can cure this by changing their diets, and balancing their progesterone, estriol, DHEA, T3, T4, and pregnenolone in addition to their testosterone.

Another study from 1998 at Hope Hospital in England (*Clinical Endocrinology* v 49) came to the same conclusions. Women with severe PMS (average age of forty) were given under-the-skin silastic implants of natural testosterone. These implants slowly release 100 mg of the hormone every six months for over two years. This is expensive and very unnecessary, but does, in fact, use natural testosterone delivered in reasonable amounts. Plasma levels rose from an average of 237 percent, which is definitely excessive. They found this regimen to be safe, and without side effects with good improvement in the short term.

Imagine the improvement if they had addressed all their basic hormones. The silastic implants are not a practical means to do this, since they need surgical implantation, are unnecessary, and very expensive. The doctors were concerned about the long term safety of low-dose androgen supplementation for women, but found, "Overall, this study provides largely reassuring data about the safety of low-dose androgen treatment in women. No patient experienced adverse symptoms while on testosterone treatment."

More and more doctors are realizing that androgens, such as DHEA, testosterone, and androstenedione are vital to the health and wellbeing of women, and are not merely "male hormones." Australian researchers (*Clinical Endocrinology & Metabolism* v 17, 2003) did a review, with many references on testosterone therapy for women. They found that "clinical symptoms of androgen insufficiency (in women) include loss of libido, diminished wellbeing, fatigue and blunted motivation and have been reported to respond well to testosterone replacement, generally without significant side effects." It is doctors like this that will help women maintain their natural hormone balance throughout life, instead of poisoning them with horse estrogen and synthetic progestins.

## ANDROGENS FOR WOMEN'S HEALTH

Finally in 2004, the medical profession provided some much needed light on the subject of androgens for female health. The entire supplement of *Mayo Clinic Proceedings* (v 79) was devoted to this subject. We will cover all five studies:

- At Columbia University, "Formulations and Use of Androgens in Women" was submitted. The authors reported that the most common symptoms of female testosterone deficiency are decreased libido and sexual pleasure, low energy and fatigue, anxiety, lack of motivation, diminished sense of wellbeing, decreased bone density, diminished muscle mass, increase in body fat, less cognitive ability, and memory loss. They recognized the need for routine measurement of free testosterone in women and supplementation when necessary. Unfortunately, they feel methyl testosterone is a valid means of administration, as well as the overpriced patches, oral salts, and injected salts. They do see promise in sublingual, vaginal, and transdermal gels, to their credit.

■ At Adult Women's Health and Medicine in Florida, an article on hot flashes was submitted. Hot flashes are all too common for premenopausal and menopausal women, especially in European countries. (This is generally not true in Asian and African countries.) Testosterone therapy is suggested for this very popular problem. Again, methyl testosterone is recommended as a valid means of administration, which shows good intentions are not always matched by intelligence, competence, or capability.

■ At the famous Mayo Clinic, bone health was studied in relation to female testosterone levels. This has already been covered in the "Osteoporosis and Bone Health" chapter. Osteoporosis is epidemic in European women, but not so much in Asian, African, or Latin women in their indigenous countries. Instead of treating bone mineral density deficiency with toxic, ineffective, expensive, and symptomatic prescription drugs, we should be doing this with natural hormones, like estriol, testosterone, and progesterone. We should also use supplements like glucosamine, minerals, flax oil, and vitamin D.

■ The fourth study, from Harvard Medical School, was "The Role of Androgens in Female Sexual Dysfunction." This has already been covered in the Female Sexuality chapter. Researchers stated that "the role of low androgen concentration in female sexual dysfunction is gaining increasing attention….and early clinical trial results suggest that they may be both effective and safe in the treatment of FSD, specifically low libido." They point out that in a survey of thousands of American women, aged eighteen to fifty-nine, (*JAMA* v 281, 1999) *a full 43 percent reported serious sexual dysfunction.* Almost half! This is a very depressing statistic that almost half of these women have serious sexual satisfaction issues. Most women keep this to themselves.

■ The last study was on safety and side effects from Johns Hopkins University. Unfortunately, it was oriented around "risks" and "side effects," instead of benefits. They pointed out that using methyl testosterone (which is still prescribed for women) and injectable salts have side effects. Real testosterone should be used, rather than nandrolone. It was admitted that transdermal gel, natural implant pellets, and patches do not have these problems. If doctors would just realize that natural testosterone, used in natural ways, in women proven to be deficient literally has *no side effects whatsoever,* and is completely safe, they would finally understand the situation. When transdermal or sublingual testosterone is used in the proper amounts, there are never any side effects. Women suffering from hyperandrogenism were also discussed. Excessive testosterone levels in women can only be lowered by diet, exercise, supplements and lifestyle, not toxic prescription drugs.

## MENOPAUSE

Some good work was done at the Kinsey Institute (*Clinical Endocrinology* v 45, 1996) on androgens in women after menopause. Women will live the last third of their lives after their menses cease. The menopausal transition is problematic for the vast majority of Western women. These problems (such as osteoporosis, memory loss, body fat, etc.) persist throughout the rest of their lives. Women forty to sixty years of age were studied to see the endocrine changes after menopause for estradiol, estrone, progesterone, LH, FSH, testosterone, androstenedione, DHEA, cortisol, and even BMI (body mass index). There were no easy answers or pat generalizations here. Each woman had a distinct and unique endocrine profile that must be addressed individually by testing each of her basic hormones.

## POST-HYSTERECTOMY

*One third of American women will needlessly suffer from a hysterectomy at an average age of only forty years.* This is somehow accepted as normal. Why do women so passively agree to be castrated for no valid reason?

Because one in three American women suffer from a hysterectomy, and their entire hormone balance upset, we need to review the few studies done on them. At McGill University in Canada (*American Journal of Obstetrics and Gynecology* v 151, 1985), women were given supplemental testosterone after hysterectomy. They were evaluated with an index of twenty-six common symptoms: "The superior efficacy of the androgen-containing preparations on somatic, psychological and total scores of the menopausal index may also be in relation to the anabolic and energizing properties of this sex steroid (testosterone)."

## PCOS IN TEENAGE GIRLS

Don't think we're just talking about older women here. Teenage girls are also strongly affected by their testosterone levels (*Endokrylogica Polska* v 52, 2001). About 70 percent of young girls have menstrual problems. Sedentary, overweight, adolescent Polish females were found to have hyper levels (2.39 nmol/l) of testosterone compared to healthy ballet dancers (1.68 nmol/l). In Italy, 23 percent of school girls were found to have hyper levels of testosterone or DHEA. 4 percent actually had Polycystic Ovarian Syndrome (PCOS) as teenagers (*JCEM* v 98, 2013). There is simply no reason to have a serious condition like PCOS at that age—or imbalanced androgens.

## CONCLUSION

Surgery and drugs are obviously not the answer for female health problems. Diet, proven supplements, natural hormone balance, avoidance of bad habits, no prescription drugs, exercise, fasting, and even meditation are the answer. *Natural health is about diet and lifestyle more than anything else.* The more women take responsibility for their own health, and stay away from doctors, the better off they will be.

As more women look at the very causes of their health problems, and not try to cover up the outward symptoms, they will be able to prevent and cure their illnesses. The medical profession is going to be decades catching up to the fact that women need youthful levels of androstenedione, DHEA, and testosterone. Any woman can basically test and balance her own hormone levels with inexpensive saliva kits without a doctor. There are almost no medical doctors or gynecologists in the world who have any ability at all to help with natural hormone testing and supplementation. Take responsibility for your own health and well-being, ladies.

# 14. Psychology and Behavior

**O**ur basic hormones have a very strong influence on our moods, outlook, and feelings of wellbeing, especially in women. There is a wealth of published information here. While going through the title of *every* single published study on women and testosterone in the last forty years in *Chemical Abstracts*, there were far, far more psychological studies on men than women. Testosterone is still considered "the male hormone." It is hard to understand why medical doctors cannot see how important testosterone is for women. We need to do such research, especially since women are more hormonally driven than men are. This has been changing in the last few years, however.

*One in four American adult women—25 percent—are taking some kind of prescription drug for a mental health condition.* This includes depression, anxiety, sleep disorders, attention problems, and outright anti-psychotic medications. 15 percent of men are also taking a psychiatric medication. Anti-psychotic medication used to be limited to mental hospitals. The use of these has risen 350 percent since the year 2000. The children, especially males, are now routinely given ADHD drugs such as Adderall®. This is plain old amphetamine! These figures are simply incomprehensible.

## DEPRESSION

Depression touches the lives of millions of American adults. Many people go undiagnosed, and therefore untreated. Depression presents itself with such classic symptoms as sadness, irritability, hopelessness, guilt, poor sleep, feelings of worthlessness, fatigue, and weight change. Hormone imbalance and depression are closely related.

- Depression in men has clearly been linked to low testosterone levels. We need to do more studies on women to see if this has the same effect on them. It most probably does. Depressed hypogonadal men should be treated with supplemental testosterone, rather than given mind numbing, dangerous, expensive, toxic psychoactive drugs with severe side effects.

- A fine study was done at the University of Connecticut in 2002 (*Journal of Gerontology* v 57A). Here, real, natural transdermal testosterone was given to hypogonadal, depressed men. Only 5 mg of testosterone per day was delivered via patches. Their free testosterone levels went from a mere 93 to 163 on the average, while estrone and estradiol were basically unchanged. That is how thorough they were. They also cited thirty-five references that demonstrated how male psychology can be impaired by low testosterone levels. They said, "Testosterone levels in older men may positively influence health perception associated with perceived physical function." This is excellent science.

- At the German Central Institute of Mental Health in 2000 (*Psychoneuroendocrinology* v 25), women aged twenty-eight to seventy-seven were studied for depression as it related to their androgen levels. They noticed, "to date, there is only sparse information about the regulation of androstenedione, testosterone and DHT (dihydrotestosterone) concentrations in women with severe major depression." What an understatement! Here, they found estradiol unrelated, but excessive levels of testosterone, androstenedione, and DHT clearly related to depression. They found generally low testosterone in the depressed women, but also hyper levels in some.

- A valuable study in 2003 from Harvard Medical School (*American Journal of Psychiatry* v 160) used natural transdermal gel in men, aged thirty to sixty-five, who suffered from depression. They were overdosed with 10 g of a one percent gel, which equates to 100 mg of actual testosterone applied to the skin and 20 mg in their blood! They also failed to measure their estrone and estradiol levels. This shows that even Harvard doctors have little basic knowledge of proper dosing. The men still responded splendidly, and largely overcame their feelings of depression. Even when given too much testosterone, the benefits were very dramatic and proven by multiple psychological testing, such as the Beck Depression Inventory, Hamilton Depression Rating Scale, and Clinical Global Impression.

■ A stunning review done at Essen University in Germany (*Maturitas* v 41, 2002) showed the same basic relationship with depression and low testosterone in women. This twenty-two page review had a full 137 cited references. Doctor Rohr is an excellent example of what progressive researchers should be doing. This also showed that excessive testosterone is related to depression (men cannot naturally have excessive levels). Women suffer from depression more than men do, so this is much more important to them. *Testosterone levels fall about 50 percent generally in women by menopause* (some women, on the other hand, suffer from androgenicity and excessive levels.)

■ Hypoandrogenism in women is related to depression, osteoporosis, low libido, genital atrophy, and higher body fat levels. In women, hyperandrogenism is related to hirstutism (body and facial hair), acne, and polycystic ovaries—which is epidemic in American women. This study further divided the women into four groups of testosterone-to-estradiol ratios for such risk categories as diabetes, CHD, and cancer. There is a wealth of information in this review that is far too comprehensive to go into in detail. This is science as it should be, with attention to women and testosterone.

■ The Rancho Bernardo Study in 1999 (*JCEM* v 84) was some of the most important research ever done, but was only concerned with men and not women. Over eight hundred hypogonadal men, over the age of fifty, had their bioavailable testosterone measured. They were then administered the Beck Depression Inventory. There was no doubt about the strong relationship between their hormone levels and states of depression: "These results suggest that testosterone treatment might improve depressed mood in older men who have low levels of bioavailable testosterone." These very same doctors should now study older women for the same phenomenon, and include other hormones such as estrone, estradiol, and estriol.

## AGGRESSIVE BEHAVIOR

There is a large volume of literature regarding aggression in both men and women. Studies indicate that there is a link between incidents of aggression and an individual's level of testosterone. Low testosterone levels show a correlation with aggressive behavior, while higher levels of testosterone tend to lessen feelings of aggression.

- A very interesting study was done at UCLA in Torrance in 1996 (*JCEM* v 81). Here, men, aged twenty-two to sixty with low testosterone were either given injections, 7.5 mg patches, or 15 mg patches. All the men generally reduced their feelings of anger, sadness, irritability, tiredness and nervousness. They increased their feelings of friendliness, good feelings, and energy. Their estradiol (E2) levels were measured before and after the administration, but they refused to reveal these levels! This is because the injections, and 15 mg patches, caused severe rises in E2.

- An impressive and extensive review was done in 2001 at the Munster University in Germany with a long list of 222 references (*European Journal of Endocrinology* v 144). Stress lowers testosterone, and stress is epidemic in Western society. Dealing properly with stress successfully allows the natural testosterone level to rise. Aggressive behavior was not shown to be caused by high testosterone levels. Even giving men excessive doses of supplemental testosterone did not increase their anger or aggression levels.

## EATING DISORDERS

Eating disorders are an epidemic in America, affecting about 30 million people. This is in addition to the obesity epidemic! This includes bulimia, binge eating, food avoidance, and anorexia nervosa. There are extreme psychiatric co-morbidities with eating disorders, including depression, suicide, anxiety, and other issues. Various illnesses and early mortality are also part of these conditions. Science has shown that, overall, hormones are unbalanced in people suffering from psychoses. Disparities in testosterone levels in particular are a contributing factor to the development of eating disorders. Anorexics, for example, show low testosterone levels. Hormone balance should be standard practice when treating eating disorders of all types.

# COGNITIVE PERFORMANCE AND ABILITIES

Research shows there is a proven relationship between testosterone levels and cognitive performance in men and women. Low testosterone levels are related to a decline in cognitive ability.

- The University of Uterect administered testosterone to young women, then studied their "spatial-location" memory and cognition. They concluded, "Testosterone has an activational effect on selective aspects of cognitive functioning." In the same journal (v 24, 1999), both men and women were studied for their spatial ability and testosterone levels: "Mental rotation scores showed a significant positive relationship with mean T levels, but not with changes in T."

- At the University of Lubeck in Germany (*Neuro-psychopharmacology* v 28, 2003), women aged forty-seven to sixty-five were given supplemental testosterone to show the effects on their "divergent and convergent" thought processes. They found that testosterone strongly affects the thought process in women, especially pre-menopausal women who have higher levels during ovulation. Here we demonstrate empirically how women are very hormonally influenced physically, mentally, and emotionally. This is why we need more knowledge about endocrine effects on their thoughts and feelings.

- The sexes are equal in intelligence, but differ in cognitive abilities. Ironically enough, when women had peak testosterone, their spatial abilities improved. With men, their spatial abilities fell during peak testosterone. At the National Institute of Aging, men were given sophisticated psychological tests. It was clear that older men, over fifty with higher testosterone, fared much better than their hypogonadal counterparts in regard to memory, stress, cognitive function, depression, and other related factors. At Leiden University in Holland, men and women with anxiety disorders were studied. Women with depression, social phobia, agoraphobia, and anxiety had lower testosterone levels. This was not found in men.

- At the University of Utah, two studies were published, including a review in 1995 complete with forty-three references (*Hormones and Behavior* v 29, and *Aggressive Behavior* v 29, 2003). They covered status,

self-regard, competitiveness, aggression, assertiveness, and dominance in young women in relation to testosterone levels. DHEA and
estradiol were not found to have any relationships to behavior in this
review. They did, however, find a definite correlation between these
factors as they relate to testosterone levels. Women with higher testosterone levels, who ranked themselves well in status, were not considered to have higher status by their peers, though.

■ One other study also showed confident, uninhibited and action-ori-
ented behavior to be correlated with higher testosterone levels in
young women. Still another study found just the opposite, however,
while others have shown no relationship at all. *There are no easy answers here.* Occupational status and testosterone in women have
shown the same inconsistencies. This is complicated by the fact that
some occupations require assertiveness, while some require other
traits. A woman lawyer or saleswoman might benefit from such behavior, while a nurse or teacher would not.

■ A study from the University of Western Ontario in 1996 (*Aggressive
Behavior* v 22) showed different results, however. Both male and female young students had their free, salivary testosterone measured.
"Within each sex, testosterone was positively correlated with aggression, and negatively correlated with pro-social personality." Men
somehow only had five times the blood testosterone level of women,
instead of the usual ten to one ratio. We all know men and women
have different cognitive abilities. Men are better with math, and
women are better with verbal skills. Musical skills are negatively correlated with testosterone in men, but positively correlated in women.
We need to study social status and testosterone in both men and
women, as there are indications this has significant relevance. Asians
generally have the highest testosterone levels, Africans moderate levels, and Europeans the lowest levels. Other aspects of this well done
review will be discussed in the appropriate chapters.

■ At the University of Michigan, men and women were studied for
the testosterone levels in association with their relationships. The researchers provided evidence that "people's orientations toward sexual relationships, in combination with their relationship status, are
associated with individual differences in testosterone." At Comenius

University in Slovakia, testosterone levels in men and women were clearly correlated with cognitive performance.

## CONCLUSION

There are a number of studies citing a correlation between levels of testosterone and behavior that we can't even begin to possibly cover. The point is made that psychology in general is strongly influenced by our endocrine systems, especially testosterone. We have enough research here to emphasize the importance of testosterone and other basic hormones. We need to apply it to real people in the everyday world. Natural hormone balance should be standard practice to treat mental and emotional issues, rather than toxic prescription drugs, which just make people worse in the end.

# 15. Obesity and BMI

**A**merica is the most overweight country in the world. Obesity rates have skyrocketed in the last thirty years from about 10 percent to 30 percent. Yes, 30 percent of adults are clinically obese. Even worse, about 18 percent of children aged six to eleven are obese. We not only eat more calories than anyone else, but more empty, nutritionless calories. We eat twice the calories we need, eight times the fat we need (42 percent of calories), twice the protein we need, insufficient fiber, 160 pounds of various sugars we don't need, and only one percent whole grains. *Overfed and undernourished.*

We should only eat two meals a day, rather than three. We also get less exercise than anyone else on earth. We don't need to wonder why we're so overweight. There are no shortcuts or "magic answers" to weight loss. Willpower is an illusion, as you can't deny the hunger instinct. The only way to lose weight and stay slim all your life is a total program of diet and lifestyle. Food, per se, doesn't make you fat; fat makes you fat. Make better food choices to stay slim while eating all you want.

*Diet is everything.* A whole grain based diet is high in nutrients, but low in calories. Worldwide studies prove the more whole grains you eat, the slimmer you'll be. In the *Journal of Nutrition* (v 139, 2009), for example, it was shown, "Higher intakes of whole grains are associated with lower total per cent body fat in adults." Diet and lifestyle are the key to staying slim all your life. *You can literally eat all you want if you eat whole, healthy, natural foods.*

## HORMONE BALANCE

Hormone balance is also critical to maintaining a healthy weight. You must have your basic hormones balanced, and testosterone is one of

the most important. Take clinically proven supplements like FOS, aci-
dophilus, flax oil, and vitamin D, especially if you're over forty. Exercise
is necessary. Going to a gym three days a week would be ideal. Even
walking the dog for a half hour every day is good. You cannot take
prescription or recreational drugs, as they upset your body and your di-
gestion. You can't have any bad habits like caffeine, alcohol, or nicotine.
Weekly fasting for twenty-four hours is a real benefit. We, of course, will
concentrate on testosterone in this chapter.

Yes, hormones do play an important part in a program of diet
and exercise. Androgen deficiency is very influential in male obesity.
Both androgen deficiency and androgen excess are very influential in
female obesity. The other major androgen is DHEA. Like testosterone,
low DHEA in men is associated with being overweight. High or low
DHEA in women causes weight problems. Low thyroid, free T3 and
T4, has dramatic effects on our body weight. You must have midrange
values for T3 and T4, and not merely be "in range." Forget your TSH
and T3 uptake.

High estrogens (estradiol and estrone) are especially important to
metabolic rate. Here, both men and women want low normal results,
and not normal ones. Why? Because Americans have excessive levels,
and what is called "normal" is really high normal. High E1 and E2 are
major causes of obesity in both sexes. The idea postmenopausal women
are "low in estrogens" is patently false. Women should have high normal estriol levels, and most all overweight women are estriol deficient.
Men do not need to test estriol.

High insulin is a very important factor as well. Your insulin level
should be about 5 IU/mL or less. Most Americans have a level twice
that. This is part of your insulin/blood sugar axis, and your blood sugar
should be 85 mg/dL or less. There are no studies on pregnenolone and
obesity, but this is part of basic hormone balance. Obese and postmenopausal women also are generally low in progesterone. Using progesterone cream is good practice. Low melatonin levels are also associated
with obesity. Growth hormone is simply too expensive ($1,800 a year), is
unstable, and requires daily injections. As usual, there was more obesity
research done on men than women. So, we will use the women's studies
that shows testosterone levels compared to their weight.

High androgens are associated with slimness in men, but with
obesity in women (*JCEM* v 100, 2015). This is especially true in

postmenopausal women. At the Clinical Hospital in Osijek (*Periodicum Biologorum* v 101, 1999), premenopausal women were found to be high in insulin, DHEA, and testosterone. At the Facharzt fur Anasthesiologie (*Obesity* v 20, 2012), overweight women were found to have excessive E1, E2, and testosterone.

Youthful testosterone levels are vital to maintaining slimness, and a low body mass index (BMI), but this is only one part of a total program of diet, exercise, and lifestyle. Expect some changes in your BMI and body fat percent from maintaining a youthful testosterone (and DHEA) level, but not any dramatic ones. Your best results will come from realizing all your hormones work together in harmony as a team. *You must balance your other basic hormones to get the most effect.*

## SCIENTIFIC FINDINGS

In recent years, researchers have begun to understand how low testosterone is related to overall health. We have established links between testosterone levels and obesity. Studies show that women who have either high or low testosterone levels can be overweight. Again, men cannot have high levels, but low levels are strongly connected with obesity. As you would expect, it is very difficult to find obesity studies on women given supplemental testosterone. Women should maintain a normal, youthful range of androgens, avoiding both hyper- and hypo-levels.

- At the University of Vienna (*Maturitas* v 29, 1998) overweight postmenopausal women low in testosterone were given topical gel. It was determined that "topically applied androgen is capable of reducing abdominal fat accumulations, as well as total body weight in postmenopausal women." Most studies, however, find overweight women to have high testosterone levels. You must be midrange. On the ZRT saliva scale, this would be about 35 on a 16 to 55 scale, for example.

- A very informative study was done at the University of Munster (*European Journal of Endocrinology* v 146, 2002). This was previously discussed in Chapter 4. Here they used oral, injected, and transdermal (patches) forms on hypogonadal men. There was very insightful information here about BMI and testosterone levels as men age. They concluded, "...testosterone appears to be an important factor contributing to these changes. Thus aging men should benefit from testosterone substitution as far as body composition is concerned." The fall in testosterone as men age was paralleled by a rise in BMI and body fat mass. This was reduced significantly by raising testosterone levels, even when using the wrong types in the wrong ways. Women have an issue with high or low androgen levels in obesity.

- At the National School of Public Health in Athens (*Annals of Nutrition and Metabolism* v 43, 1999), healthy elderly men were studied for their body mass and their hormone levels. Not surprisingly, they found that low testosterone was equated with obesity, and high testosterone equated with slimness. They also found higher estradiol levels equated with obesity, and low estradiol with slimness. They also found the more dietary saturated fat the men ate, the lower their testosterone.

- At the University of Pennsylvania School of Medicine (*JCEM* v 84, 1999), elderly men were given real transdermal testosterone. Of course, all of these men were low in testosterone, since they were all over the age of sixty-five. This was a true double blind study, where half the men were given placebo patches. This lasted a full three years. The men lost an average of almost seven pounds of body fat, while making no changes at all in their diet or lifestyle. They gained almost five pounds of real muscle. When you lose fat and gain muscle, your total body mass is exponentially improved. This was all done by simply raising their testosterone naturally to youthful levels, and not asking them to do anything else at all. Imagine what they could have done with more hormone balance, a better diet, and some reasonable exercise!

- In a rare study of women at the University of Alabama (*JCEM* v 85, 2000), they found youthful testosterone levels in postmenopausal women were correlated with slimness, and "total lean mass and leg lean mass were significantly correlated with free testosterone." Remember that we are talking about the normal ranges for postmenopausal women for free testosterone, and the women in the higher normal ranges were slimmer, and had more lean muscle mass and less fat mass. Women who have hyper levels of testosterone and DHEA outside of the normal range have a condition called "androgenicity," and need to lower those levels.

- Anorexic women are low in testosterone, estradiol, T3, and T4 (*Hormone Metabolism Research* v 27, 1995). Diabetic women tend to be high in testosterone, as are those with breast cancer, PCOS, hirstutism, and other conditions.

## MAINTAINING A HEALTHY WEIGHT

People endlessly look for Magic Weight Loss Supplements, but *only diet and lifestyle will keep you slim and healthy.* You can eat all you want and be slim if you just make better food choices. The following figures (below and on the next page) show the average body fat percentage of women and men, respectively, as they age.

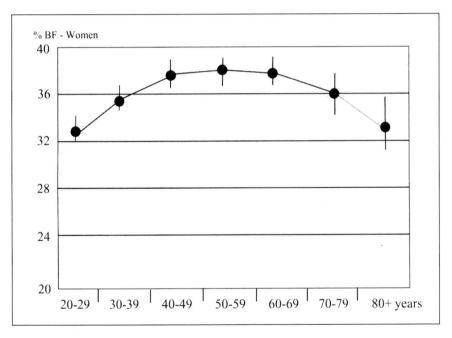

**Figure 15.1.** Female Body Fat Percentage

Ironically, we have lower body fat in our eighties. But this certainly isn't due to good diet and exercise! Women average about 34 percent body fat, while men average about 23 percent. Women therefore maintain about 50 percent more adipose tissue. You can see by the above charts how body fat rises in both American men and women

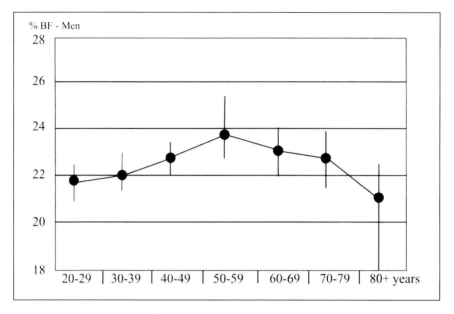

**Figure 15.2.** Male Body Fat Percentage

until about the age of sixty. After the age of sixty it falls, due to failing health and the inability of the body to maintain itself. Such muscle loss is called "sarcopenia."

You can avoid this with a total program of holistic health. Americans are literally the fattest people on earth, as you can see by the above charts. You'll find that people in Third World countries will have about one third less fat on their bodies due to less food available, lower calorie intake, less animal foods available, and harder physical work that is required to survive.

## CONCLUSION

Obviously, we need more research with regard to women. The same advice on diet and lifestyle applies for maintaining slimness, as in every other chapter in this book. Men need to keep the youthful levels of testosterone they enjoyed at about the age of thirty. Women need to keep the youthful levels while avoiding excessive ones. You must balance your other basic hormone levels (see Chapter 17 for more about this) for optimum benefits.

# 16. Exercise and Strength

**Y**outhful testosterone levels make us stronger and help maintain muscle mass. When and how you exercise has an effect on your testosterone. Use resistance training as well as aerobic exercise to help keep your testosterone and DHEA higher naturally.

The bottom line is that exercise helps *normalize* hormone levels, and that certainly includes testosterone. *Exercise helps normalize your hormones.* This is especially true with women, since they can have excessive as well as deficient levels. Having balanced hormone levels makes us stronger and gives us more endurance as well. One major reason that Americans have such out-of-sync hormone levels is our extreme inactivity. Regular exercise will help lower excessive hormone levels and raise deficient ones.

## SCIENTIFIC FINDINGS

As expected, there is a large body of research regarding the effect of exercise on male testosterone levels, but very little on females.

- At the National Institutes of Health (*American Journal of Physiology* v 283, 2002) the doctors examined testosterone in men in a study titled, "Free Testosterone Index with Fat Free Mass and Strength in Aging Men." They found higher testosterone levels were very good predictors of muscle strength in men ranging in age from twenty-four to ninety: "Muscle mass and strength losses during aging may be associated with declining levels of serum testosterone in men." They found also that the men with higher testosterone had more strength, muscle mass, and less body fat. This was a most detailed and sophisticated study with fifty references.

- In the same journal (v 282, 2002), doctors at the University of Texas gave hypogonadal men injections of salts. Despite using the wrong dose in the wrong way, they still elicited results in six months: "Older men receiving testosterone increased total leg lean body mass, muscle volume, and leg and arm muscle strength." Imagine the results they would have gotten from using proper doses of sublingual or transdermal testosterone.

- The doctors at UCLA in Torrance (*JCEM* v 85, 2000) were sophisticated enough to use transdermal gel in men. They found the usual increases in fat free mass, decreases in body fat, and impressive increases in strength and muscle size by also having the men exercise. The doctors stated that "mean muscle strength in the leg press exercise increases by 11 to 13 kg in all treatment groups by ninety days. Moderate increases were also observed in arm/chest muscle strength." This is good science by good researchers.

- More modern doctors at the University of Connecticut (*Journals of Gerontology* v 56A, 2001) used transdermal testosterone patches (5 mg delivered daily) on elderly men (average age seventy-six) for one year. Estrogen (estradiol and estrone) levels, PSA levels, and prostate volume basically remained the same. Their free, unbound levels of testosterone rose 75 percent, resulting in a 38 percent increase in strength. Body fat decreased significantly, while lean body mass (muscle) increased, as did bone mineral density. Many other biological parameters were measured, and this was a very professional long term study. More good science.

- It is proven that exercise will help improve, normalize, and balance your hormone levels. If you exercise regularly *you will make permanent changes,* as long as you continue your program. At the University of Kanazawa, in Japan, (*Horumon to Rinsho* v 40, 1992), young men (average age of twenty-four) exercised vigorously on stationary bicycles. *Their growth hormone went up an amazing 1,850 percent!* Their parathyroid hormone went up 182 percent. Their testosterone went up a full 110 percent, or more than double. Vitamin D3, free T3, and free T4 all doubled. Insulin and C-reactive peptide both fell. This was an exceptionally intricate and unique study where dozens of such parameters were studied. Fine science here.

- Studies at the University of Texas (*Journal of Laboratory and Clinical Medicine* v 34, 1999) found strength benefits from both supplemental testosterone and growth hormone (rhGH). The researchers summarized that "testosterone administration to human patients will increase muscle strength and muscle protein synthesis and may stimulate intramuscular IFG-1 system. rhGH administration to human patients will improve muscle strength in GH-deficient adults and improve body composition in older individuals and GH-deficient adults."

- Fortunately, at the University of Jyvaskyla, in Finland, (*Acta Physiologica Scandinavia* v 148, 1993) women were included in studies! Testosterone tends to fall in women as they age, especially prior to menopause. Researchers found that "In the females, significant positive correlations were observed between the individual values in serum testosterone concentration and the values both in the muscle cross sectional area (CSA) and in maximal force (physical strength). The present results imply that the decreasing basic level of blood testosterone over the years in aging people, especially in females, may lead to decreasing anabolic effects on muscles, thus having an association with age-related declines in the maximal voluntary neuromuscular performance capacity in aging people."

  They said further, "In the female subjects, the individual values in serum testosterone correlated significantly with the individual values of maximal force, and with the individual values of maximal rate of force production, as well as with the individual values of the CSA of older females."

- The next year (*Acta Physiologica Scandinavia* v 150), a similar study was done. Serum testosterone went up, and cortisol fell, in both sexes during the twelve week training. "The present findings demonstrate that considerable gains may take place in strength during progressive strength training both in middle-aged and elderly people." The findings also point out the importance of the anabolic hormonal level for the trainability of muscle strength of an individual during prolonged strength training especially in elderly males and females."

■ At the Polish Academy of Sciences (*Endokrynoliga Polska* v 52, 2001), young girls aged sixteen to nineteen were compared as to exercise and profiles of eight hormones. Menstrual problems occur in about 70 percent of adolescents. The ballet dancers were much healthier overall than the sedentary girls. They had less menstrual and other health issues. The sedentary girls had higher LH, prolactin, estradiol, and testosterone levels. The sedentary girls were given a four month exercise program, which improved their hormonal profile and their monthly problems. The conclusion was, "Moderate physical activity is recommended for the therapy of menstrual disorders." It is obvious we need more research on teenage girls and their hormones.

■ The scientists at Pennsylvania State University also realized testosterone is important for women (*European Journal of Applied Physiology* v 78, 1998). Untrained women were given a three stage program of resistance exercise (weight lifting). Testosterone and growth hormone went up in the women, while cortisol fell. The authors stated, "These data illustrate that untrained individuals may exhibit early-phase endocrine adaptations during a resistance training program. These hormonal adaptations may influence and help to mediate other adaptations in the nervous system and muscle fibers." Research such as this shows women as well as men normalize and improve their entire endocrine balance with regular exercise in a very short time.

■ Female adolescent athletes were studied at Southeastern Lousiana University (*European Journal of Applied Physiology* v 86, 2001). "It appears therefore, that DHEA, testosterone, and leptin concentrations increase in response to running in adolescent female runners. Data also suggest that training and/or maturation increases resting testosterone concentrations and testosterone responses to running in adolescent female runners during a training session." Again, exercise improves the hormonal profile in women of all ages, including teenagers.

## CONCLUSION

We have seen how scant the research is for women, and there is no reason to go on with the hundreds of studies for men. Regular exercise is important to maintaining hormonal balance. Exercise will help lower those that are too high and raise those that are too low. If you are low in any hormones, it is not enough to simply take a supplement. Life extension means living a healthy lifestyle, not just taking hormone supplements. You must eat well, exercise regularly, and avoid bad habits (such as caffeine and alcohol) that will unbalance your endocrine system. Maintaining youthful levels of all your basic hormones will make you more physically fit, and give you more endurance and strength throughout your life.

# 17. Your Other Hormones

**M**en need to balance their basic eleven hormones as much as possible in order to prevent and cure illness, enjoy full health, and have long life. Women need to monitor their estriol levels as well. If there is one basic thing to repeat over and over, it is that all *our hormones work together as a team in concert*, and they all must be at youthful levels as much as possible. Do not just be concerned with testosterone or any other hormone by itself without including all the others that work together with it.

The twelve basic hormones are:

- DHEA
- Estradiol
- Estriol
- Estrone
- Growth Hormone
- Insulin
- Melatonin
- Pregnenolone
- Progesterone
- T3
- T4
- Testosterone

## DHEA

DHEA is a very important, basic, and powerful androgen. The benefits of having a youthful DHEA level are far too numerous to mention. There are hundreds of impressive published clinical studies in men and women of all ages. Many of these studies, however, did not measure the patients to see if they were deficient. People were often given excessive 50 mg or higher doses, even the women! *Women need half the DHEA men do.* Such irresponsible science is simply inexcusable.

Women have lower levels of DHEA and need to take less as a supplement. Never, never take DHEA without first testing your blood (either free DHEA or DHEA-S) or saliva levels to see if you are deficient. Our levels usually start to fall about the age of forty, and keep falling until we die. Some older people, especially women, can have high-normal or even hyper DHEA levels as they age. Thus, you cannot just assume you are deficient because you are forty or older. Men can take 25 mg daily if they are low, and check their level after six months to see if this is the correct dose. Women can take 12.5 mg (half tablets), and check their level the same way. Do not accept a normal level for your age, but rather keep *the youthful level* you had about the age of thirty.

## PREGNENOLONE

Pregnenolone is the basic source of all the other sex hormones, but is the "forgotten" or "orphan" hormone, because we know so little about it. This is *the* basic brain, memory, learning and cognition hormone, yet there has been almost no research done on it. What knowledge we do have is overwhelmingly positive, and shows great promise for supplementation in people who need it. Doctors do not know nor care about pregnenolone—this includes endocrinologists and neurologists, amazingly enough.

Our levels generally fall at about the age of thirty-five or forty for both men and women, and then stabilize and remain low. Men over the age of forty can take 50 mg a day, and check their levels after, say, six months. Women over forty can take 25 mg a day, and do the same check. Taking 100 mg of PS (phosphatidyl serine) along with your pregnenolone is an effective way of avoiding senility, memory loss, impaired cognition, and Alzheimer's.

## MELATONIN

Melatonin is truly a miraculous hormone that regulates our biological aging clock. The media will tell you this is merely good for jet lag! The truth is that melatonin is being studied for cancer prevention and treatment, among many other benefits. Our melatonin levels fall from the time we leave our teenage years, and keep falling until we die.

A good dose is 1.5 mg (half tabs) for women, and 3 mg for men, if you are over forty. You can test your levels (at 3:00 AM with saliva) after, say, six months to see if this is the correct dose. Some people have naturally high levels, and cannot take melatonin until they reach their fifties or sixties, so be sure to test your level. Some life extension advocates advise taking large doses of 5 and 10 mg, which is very irresponsible. As always, we are looking for youthful levels, and not high, out-of-range results.

## ESTRIOL

Estriol (E3) is the "forgotten," good, or beneficial estrogen. There is very, very little published information on estriol, amazingly enough. This is *the* most abundant estrogen in both men and women, comprising 80 to 90 percent of human estrogen. Yet, we know little about it, and almost nothing regarding men. Fortunately, very few men have been found to have either high or low estriol levels. What we do know is most impressive regarding benefits for women.

Doctors, gynecologists, and endocrinologists generally do not know, nor care, about this most abundant and basic estrogen. No United States pharmaceutical corporation makes an estriol product, and no chain or independent pharmacies carry estriol in any form. The very few doctors who do know about it are so ignorant they generally recommend toxic, unnatural oral estriol ester salts. You can find good, inexpensive estriol creams on the Internet for $20. You need 0.3 percent, or 200 mg of estriol, per 2 ounce jar. Use a half gram daily. This will apply 1.5 mg on the skin, and 0.5 mg (30 percent) should be absorbed. Sublingual estriol vegetable oil solution (500 mcg per drop) would be another natural and effective means of delivery. A compounding pharmacist would charge you probably $50 for $1 worth of estriol. A DMSO solution could also be made (500 mcg per drop), but is not legally available. For either, just add one gram of estriol to 16 ml (500 drops) of vegetable oil, or 99 percent DMSO.

There is not one single published study in the scientific literature that has measured women of different ages for their estriol level, and made a chart showing normal levels! This is beyond understanding for the most basic of all human estrogens. Rural Asian, macrobiotic, and vegetarian women have higher levels on the average. Your doctor will not know anything about estriol, but can send in a blood sample to a major lab and get your *free* (not bound) estriol (you must emphasize this) level checked. It is much easier and cheaper to just saliva test your level.

# ESTRONE

Estrone (E1) is a powerful and potentially dangerous estrogen. Men over fifty literally have higher estrone (and estradiol) levels than their post-menopausal wives! This is frightening! Estrone deficiency in men seems almost non-existent. Western women are generally excessive in estrone (and estradiol), and rarely deficient. However, women with hysterectomies (one third of American women) sometimes have a problem, since their ovaries have atrophied and died, even if they were not removed. One third of American women will, in fact, get castrated.

You can test your free (you must emphasize this), not bound, estrone level with a blood draw, or use a saliva test. Men and women want *low normal levels*, not midrange levels. Deficient women can use a naturally synthesized, bioidentical sublingual estrone, patch, or cream, but *never equine (horse) estrogen or oral tablets*. Use a compounding pharmacist, even though you'll be overcharged. On the ZRT saliva scale, a 1.3 level is ideal for men and postmenopausal women. You cannot buy estrone creams online.

# ESTRADIOL

Estradiol (E2) is the most powerful and most dangerous estrogen, and the least abundant percentage-wise. Estradiol deficiency in men seems almost non-existent. Women are rarely deficient in estradiol. Western women are generally excessive as just mentioned. However, after a hysterectomy, there may be a deficiency of estradiol. Like estrone, men and women want *low normal levels*, and not midrange. Deficient women can use a naturally synthesized, bioidentical form, just as with estrone. *Never use equine (horse) estrogen or oral tablets*. On the ZRT saliva scale, a 0.5 level is ideal for men and postmenopausal women.

# PROGESTERONE

Progesterone is needed by both men and women. This is not a "feminizing" hormone for men. On the contrary, it opposes and balances the estrogens in both sexes. Saliva testing does not work, as this is a fat soluble hormone. Just find a good, reliable brand of transdermal progesterone cream that contains 1,000 mg per 2 ounce jar (500 mg per ounce). You can get these online for $10. For women, this is covered in my book, *Natural Health for Women*. They can use this according to their menopausal status. Men can simply use one eighth teaspoon five days a week directly on their scrotum. This is covered in my book, *The Natural Prostate Cure*. You really do not need to get a blood test for this.

## THYROID

Thyroid problems are epidemic in America, and usually the problem is lack of hormones (hypothyroidism) rather than excessive (hyperthyroidism) ones. *T4* (L-thyroxine or Synthroid®) is usually low rather than *T3* (triiodothyronine or Cytomel®). Contrary to the usual wisdom, both Synthroid and Cytomel are synthesized, but bio-identical hormones, chemically identical to the ones in your body. Often naïve and uneducated naturopathic doctors will recommend Armour Thyroid, which is derived from bovine (cow) or porcine (pig) thyroid glands. Do not use this, as it has a four to one mixture of L-thyroxine and triiodothyronine. Therefore, the only people who can use this are the rare (5 percent) ones who are low in both.

Saliva kits are not currently available, but should be. You can get home blood spot kits for $75. In the United States, go to www.walkinlab.com for a real $90 blood test without a doctor. You can overpay a doctor and get a blood draw for free T3 and free T4. Do *not* let the doctor waste your time and money testing your TSH, T3 uptake, or other unnecessary tests. Just get your free T3 and free T4 measured.

Do not accept low normal ranges, even though your doctor may tell you this is "fine" as long as you are in range. You want a healthy, *youthful* midrange level. If you are low in T4, try 50 mcg of generic Levoxyl. If you are low in T3, try 12.5 mcg of generic Tiromel. If this isn't enough, then use more, but be careful. You can buy these legally and inexpensively from the Mexican online pharmacies without a prescription. If you are low, you will probably get the most dramatic and obvious effects with thyroid hormones than any others.

## GROWTH HORMONE

Growth hormone (somatatropin) falls as we age, and almost disappears in the elderly. There are no saliva tests for GH, and you *cannot* use IGF-1 levels, contrary to the popular wisdom. IGF-1 does not parallel GH, no matter what you read somewhere else. GH levels vary during the day, so the only accurate way to measure it is four blood draws three hours hours apart in a clinic. If you are over fifty, you most probably are deficient and can use a supplement.

*No OTC growth hormone supplements work.* Period. Write this down somewhere so you don't forget it. Everything you see sold in health food stores, in catalogs, and on the Internet have no value whatsoever, regardless of how well the advertising is written. The homeopathic GH is the worst fraud. Only real prescription, injectable rhGH (recombinant human) works. The problem is not only the fact it has to be injected subcutaneously (under the skin and not in your veins), but that it will cost you a minimum of $1,800 a year for Chinese GH.

You need 1 UI daily, which is 30 IU (10 mg) of rhGH every month. American brands will cost you about $3,600 a year minimum. Chinese GH was available from the foreign online pharmacies legally, but this has been stopped by customs. All the inexpensive and exotic peptides like hexarelin have failed for one reason or another. We are years away from inexpensive GH, such as veterinarians use for cows. Unless you're willing to pay $1,800 a year and inject it daily, you simply cannot use this. Sublingual use in DMSO may well be possible, but there is no science here yet. GH is totally overrated merely due to its expense; it is hard to synthesize the 198 amino acid chain.

## INSULIN

Insulin has to be blood tested. You can use online labs without a doctor. You want a level of 4 to 5 IU/ml. You can also your insulin *response* with a GTT (glucose tolerance test). For a GTT, you simply drink a cup of glucose, and your blood sugar is measured two hours later. If your fasting blood sugar is 85 or less, you probably don't need to bother. You can also buy blood spot HbA1c tests at any drug store. This is a six month average of your glycation. Look for a 4.7 level, not the accepted level.

Americans have an epidemic of blood sugar problems, especially insulin resistance, metabolic syndrome, diabetes, and hypoglycemia. "Insulin resistance" means our body no longer responds well to insulin, so we produce higher amounts in order to compensate. Testing your insulin per se may not tell you much. If you are insulin resistant, or have any blood sugar dysmetabolism, you have to change your diet and lifestyle. As long as your pancreas is intact, this can be very easy to do—with very fast results. You must cut down on meat and fats, take dairy out of your life, not eat refined grains, and eat no fruit, sugars or sweeteners whatsoever. This includes honey, molasses, stevia, fruit juice, etc. There are a variety of supplements that will help, including lipoic acid, CoQ10, beta glucan, and a complete mineral supplement.

## CORTISOL

Cortisol is the stress hormone. The only way to test this is to do a four sample 12 hour saliva profile at 9/1/5/9. If you are too low or too high, then only better diet, exercise, ceasing bad habits, and a general change in lifestyle is going to help you. You must change your diet and lifestyle and deal with whatever stress is causing this. Balancing your other hormones will go a long way towards normalizing your cortisol levels. *This is completely optional, and you don't need to bother with cortisol at all.*

## CONCLUSION

All your basic hormones should be balanced, as they all work together in harmony, as a team. Raising your testosterone when some of your other hormones are deficient is just not going to give you the effects you want or can get. It may seem arduous to try and test all your basic hormones and balance them, but the more you do, the more benefits you will get. All can be saliva tested very inexpensively, except for growth hormone and progesterone. All are available legally under United States Code Section 21, Section 331 for personal use (up to fifty dosage units) imported by mail or coming back into the country in person.

# 18. Seven Steps to Natural Health

**W**ith these seven steps, you can cure "incurable" illnesses like cancer, diabetes, heart disease and others naturally without drugs, surgery, or chemotherapy. There are seven vital steps to take if you want optimum health and long life. Do your best to do all of them.

**1.** American macrobiotic whole grain-based diet is central to everything. Diet cures disease; everything else is secondary.

**2.** Proven supplements are powerful when you're eating right. There are only about eighteen scientifically proven supplements for those over forty, and eight for those under forty.

**3.** Natural hormone balance is the third step. The basic hormones are listed on page 101. You can do this inexpensively without a doctor.

**4.** Exercise is vital, even if it is just a half hour of walking a day. Whether it is aerobic or resistance, you need to exercise regularly.

**5.** Fasting is the most powerful healing method known to man. Just fast from dinner to dinner on water one day a week. Join our monthly Young Again two day fast on the last weekend of every month. The fasting calendar is at www.youngagain.org.

**6.** No prescription drugs, except *temporary* antibiotics or pain medication during an emergency. The only exception is insulin for type 1 diabetics who have no operant pancreas.

**7.** The last step is to limit or end any bad habits such as alcohol, coffee, recreational drugs, or desserts. You don't have to be a saint, but you do have to be sincere.

The only step to add would be affirmative prayer or meditation. Faith will move mountains.

# Recommended Reading

Hufnagel, Vicki G. with Susan, K. Golant, *No More Hysterectomies.* Mass Paperback, 1995.

West, Stanley, MD and Paula Dranov, *The Hysterectomy Hoax.* Next Decade Inc., 2002

Stokes, Naomi, M., *The Castrated Woman.* Frankling Watts, 1986.

# About the Author

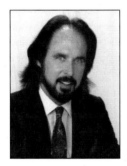

*Roger Mason* is an internationally known research chemist who studies natural health and life extension. He develops unique natural supplements and products. He writes books, articles, speaks to groups, and has an Internet site. Roger has opened up a charitable trust, the Young Again Foundation, and continues to pursue his research in the many areas of natural health and healing. This is his tenth book on natural health. You can go to his website at www.youngagain.org to get his free weekly newsletter and over three hundred articles on natural health. Roger and his wife live in Wilmington, NC.

# Index

# Other Square One Titles of Interest

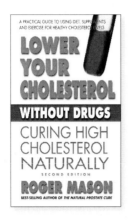

## Lower Your Cholesterol Without Drugs
### SECOND EDITION

Curing High Cholesterol Naturally

Roger Mason

Research shows that high cholesterol is a major risk factor for coronary heart disease. While prescription drugs can lower cholesterol, they come with many unwelcome side effects. In *Lower Your Cholesterol Without Drugs,* Roger Mason offers you a safe, effective way to treat this condition and improve your health. The book looks at the causes of high cholesterol and then explains how a balanced, vitamin-rich diet can naturally enhance your well-being.

$9.95 US • 128 pages • 6 x 9-inch paperback • ISBN 978-0-7570-0367-7

## The Natural Diabetes Cure
### SECOND EDITION

Curing Blood Sugar Disorders Without Drugs

Roger Mason

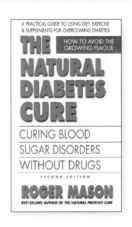

In *The Natural Diabetes Cure,* Roger Mason provides an effective nutritional approach to preventing and combating type 2 diabetes. The book describes how diabetes develops, and then explains how a balanced diet of whole grains, healthy fats, and fresh vegetables can greatly improve overall health and well-being. Additional chapters discuss vitamins and nutritional supplements that can help regulate blood sugar, and offer other strategies for leading a longer, higher-quality life.

$9.95 • 128 pages • 6 x 9-inch paperback • ISBN 978-0-7570-0369-1

# Lower Blood Pressure Without Drugs

## SECOND EDITION

Curing Your Hypertension Naturally

Roger Mason

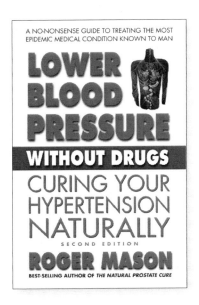

Over sixty-five million Americans have high blood pressure, which is defined as 140/90. Over forty million more are pre-hypertensive, with blood pressures reaching 120/80. High blood pressure can cause strokes, heart attacks, and congestive heart failure. Although prescription drugs may effectively lower blood pressure, they have potentially very dangerous side effects. Fortunately, there are natural alternatives to lowering blood pressure and preventing these serious health conditions. In this updated edition of *Lower Blood Pressure Without Drugs,* best-selling author Roger Mason provides a proven nutritional approach to lowering blood pressure safely and naturally.

The book begins by explaining what hypertension is, what causes it, and how it is diagnosed. From there, it goes on to describe how a simple diet, rich in whole grains and low in fat, can improve both blood pressure and general health. This is followed by chapters that address such key topics as the best nutritional supplements to take; which exercises are most effective; how to maintain hormonal balance; and, just as important, how to overcome poor dietary and lifestyle habits. Also included is a scientifically valid diet and exercise program that is easy to follow and incorporate into your lifestyle.

You have the power to avoid becoming a walking time bomb. Be good to yourself. Take the first steps towards safely and effectively lowering your blood pressure with *Lower Blood Pressure Without Drugs.*

$9.95 US • 128 pages • 6 x 9-inch paperback •
ISBN 978-0-7570-0366-0

# The Natural Prostate Cure

## THIRD EDITION

A Practical Guide to Using Diet and
Supplements for a Healthy Prostate

Roger Mason

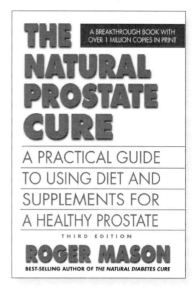

By age fifty, three out of four men have
enlarged prostates, which can lead to
serious health problems, and one in
three men has cancer cells in his prostate.
Traditional treatments for the more critical
of these prostate-related illnesses include
surgery, radiation, chemotherapy, and even
castration. These methods are dangerous
and have potentially drastic results. Worst
of all, they fail to address the real cause of
prostate problems.

In this updated 3rd edition of *The Natural Prostate Cure,* author Roger
Mason provides a unique and effective alternative to risky prostate
surgery and drug therapies. Based upon years of research by Mason
and his peers, this essential book explains how most prostate problems
originate from poor nutrition. The book opens with a basic lesson in
proper diet and presents the best supplements for maintaining a healthy
prostate, including beta-sitosterol, a vital key to prostate well-being.
The author then talks about steps that can be taken to cure prostate
disease, including cancer. Finally, the author discusses how hormone
imbalances--caused largely by poor diet--are a major factor contributing
to prostate issues. The last chapters of the book suggest hormone
treatments that can prevent and combat these potentially serious conditions.

You don't have to undergo life-threatening surgery or take dangerous drugs
to maintain a healthy prostate. With *The Natural Prostate Cure,* you will
discover how to treat prostate problems safely, effectively, and naturally.

$9.95 US • 144 pages • 6 x 9-inch paperback • ISBN 978-0-7570-0476-6

# For more information about our books,
## visit our website at www.squareonepublishers.com